Earl Mindell's
SOY MIRACLE

Earl Mindell, R.Ph., Ph.D.

A FIRESIDE BOOK
Published by Simon & Schuster
New York   London   Toronto   Sydney   Tokyo   Singapore

FIRESIDE
Rockefeller Center
1230 Avenue of the Americas
New York, New York 10020

FIRESIDE and colophon are registered trademarks
of Simon & Schuster Inc.

Designed by Richard Oriolo

Manufactured in the United States of America

10 9 8 7 6 5

Library of Congress Cataloging-in-Publication Data
Mindell, Earl.
    Earl Mindell's soy miracle / Earl Mindell.
        p.   cm.
    "A Fireside book".
    Includes bibliographical references and index.
    1. Soyfoods—Therapeutic use.   2. Cookery (Soybeans)
I. Title.
    RM666.S59M55   1995
    613.2'6—dc20   94-24766
                                                        CIP

ISBN: 0-671-89820-5

The ideas, procedures, and suggestions contained in this book are
not intended to replace the services of a trained health professional.
All matters regarding your health require medical supervision. You
should consult your physician before adopting the procedures in this
book. Any applications of the treatments set forth in this book are at
the reader's descretion.

Acknowledgments

I wish to express my deep and lasting appreciation to the people who have assisted me in this book, especially Bonny Redlich, a superb researcher; Judith Eaton, M.S., R.D., and Karen Lefkowitz, M.S., for their wonderful recipes; Sherry Wehner of Protein Technologies, Int., St. Louis; the Soyfoods Association of America and the United Soybean Board for their help; and all the soyfood producers mentioned in this book. In addition, I would like to thank all of the soybean researchers in the United States and throughout the world from whose work we all benefit. Finally, special thanks to Josh Gerber for his fine proofreading, to my editors Marilyn Abraham and Sheila M. Curry for their wise advice and assistance, and to Philip Metcalf and Carole Berglie for their help with copyediting and production. Much thanks to Richard Curtis, my agent, for his help throughout the years.

Contents

PART IV GET MORE SOY IN YOUR LIFE!

PART V SEVENTY SUPER SOY RECIPES

Part I

SOY: THE MIRACLE FOOD

One

The Soy Story: Explaining the Miracle

In February 1994, some 250 scientists, nutritionists, and health-care professionals gathered in Mesa, Arizona, to hear the latest findings on the prevention and treatment of cancer and heart disease. The group included researchers from the Hirosaki University School of Medicine in Japan, the University of Helsinki in Finland, and the University of Milan in Italy. They were joined by colleagues from major U.S. research organizations, including the National Cancer Institute and the Harvard School of Public Health. Heart specialists reported on a groundbreaking treatment for lowering cholesterol that is as effective as medication but without any unpleasant or dangerous side effects. Cancer researchers talked about special compounds that can inhibit enzymes that stimulate tumor growth, deactivate potent hormones that can promote cancer, and normalize cancer cells. What made this conference unique is that these scientists were not talking about some fantastic drug of the future or some rare chemical. They were talking about a foodstuff that is harvested in vast amounts in the United States and that is inexpensive and readily available at supermarkets and natural food stores. They were talking about soybeans and soybean products.

In recent years, scientists have isolated compounds in plant foods—phytochemicals—that may protect against disease in a variety of ways. Some can lower cholesterol levels, thus reducing the risk of heart disease. Others are antioxidants that protect cells from free radicals—unstable oxygen molecules that can damage normal cells. Still others can deactivate carcinogens (cancer-causing substances) or boost the immune system, enhancing the body's ability to ward off infection. Scientists have dubbed these plant chemicals *nutriceuticals* because of their potential health benefits.

It's not surprising that plants would be such a rich source of healthful compounds. Centuries before the age of antibiotics, natural healers and herbalists used plants to treat a wide variety of illnesses. In fact, nearly half of all the thousands of drugs that are commonly used and prescribed today are either derived from a plant source or are chemical imitations of a plant compound.

Soybeans in particular are abundant in many different types of phytochemicals, some of which are unique to this food. They include:

- **Isoflavones**—Compounds that are similar to natural estrogen but with one important difference: these plant estrogens may help prevent hormone-dependent cancers. (Some scientists believe that they may even prevent hot flashes in menopausal women!)

- **Genistein**—A compound that may stop the spread of some forms of cancer at its earliest stages, and may even help to prevent heart disease. Researchers are investigating genistein as a treatment for prostate cancer.

- **Protease Inhibitors**—Described by one researcher as a "universal anti-carcinogen," these compounds may block the action of cancer-causing enzymes.

- **Phytic Acids**—Compounds that have been shown to inhibit the growth of tumors in laboratory animals.

Although much more research needs to be done, and much about soy still needs to be learned, many leading scientists agree that there is strong evidence that soy may protect against cancer and other diseases that are virtual epidemics in the West. Soy's possible role as a cancer fighter has attracted the attention of the National Cancer Institute, which has given top priority to investigating the role of soy as a potential protector against many forms of cancer.

The Asian Advantage

Although the United States is the world's leading producer of soybeans, Americans are not the world's leading consumers of this food. Far from it: half of the U.S. soy crop is shipped overseas and most of what is kept is used to make cooking oil or animal feed. In many parts of Asia, however, soy foods are a dietary staple. For example, the average Japanese person consumes 50 to 80 grams (roughly 2 to 3 ounces) of soy food daily, in many different forms ranging from traditional bean curd or tofu to miso—a bean paste used for seasoning and in soups—to soy milk—a delicious beverage. In contrast, the average American eats a minuscule 5 grams of soy food daily, mostly in the form of oil hidden in foods such as margarine, salad dressings, and baked goods or as protein extenders in processed foods such as frozen dinners or diet drinks.

Does eating soy foods really make a difference? Judge for yourself by comparing Japanese and American health:

1. Japanese people have the longest life span of any nationality.

2. The Japanese have much lower rates of colon cancer and lung cancer than Americans.

3. Japan has the lowest rate of death from heart disease for men in the world, and the second lowest for women.

4. American women are four times more likely to die from breast cancer than Japanese women.

5. American men are five times more likely to die from prostate cancer than Japanese men.

Although the Japanese diet contains other foods that may offer protection against disease—for example, it tends to be lower in fat and higher in fiber than Western cuisine—many scientists believe that frequent consumption of soy foods is a major factor in Japanese health and longevity. Many researchers also believe that simply by adding as little as 2 ounces of soy food daily in an already healthful diet will provide Westerners with protection against "Western diseases" such as cancer and heart disease.

In *Earl Mindell's Soy Miracle,* I review what I've learned from interviews with leading scientists who are researching the various compounds in soy, and from analyzing the hundreds of scientific articles that have been written about this amazing food.

Earl Mindell's Soy Miracle will introduce Westerners to the potential benefits of soy foods, and show how easy it is to incorporate soy foods into your daily diet. For example, we all have seen tofu in Japanese and Chinese restaurants and even in supermarkets, but few of us know what to do with it. This book will introduce you to the many different soy products that are readily available in grocery and natural food stores, and will explain how they can become an important—and enjoyable—part of your daily menu. I will show you how some soy products can serve as tasty and healthful substitutes for fatty foods such as cream, meat, and cheese. I will show you how soy foods can be incorporated into virtually any cuisine, from Italian to Tex-Mex. I will show you how soy products can be used to make luscious creamy desserts and shakes that are virtually fat-free and healthful. I will show you how you can get more soy in your life without giving up the foods or flavors that you enjoy. I consulted with dieticians and cooks who are specialists in using soy foods, and they have provided the recipes in this book.

Although soy may be a wonder food, it is still only one food that should be included in a varied, well-balanced diet. When appropriate, I discuss other foods and nutrients that along with soy can promote better health.

Soy Through the Ages

- The Chinese were the first to use soybeans as food. Legend has it, around 1500 B.C. two Chinese warlords got hopelessly lost in a northern Chinese desert. Starving, they survived by eating the hard "peas," or seeds, from soybeans. By around 1100 B.C., soybeans were being cultivated in east-central China and soon became a staple of the Chinese diet. The Chinese showed their high regard for the soybean by naming it *ta tou,* which means "greater bean."

- Bean curd made from soybeans (known as tofu) has been used for several centuries in traditional Chinese medicine. Externally, it was placed on sores and ulcers to promote healing; internally, it was used in hot soups to treat colds.

- The soybean was introduced to Japan around 100 A.D. and soon spread throughout other Asian countries. Although the Chinese may have been the first to use soy, the Japanese were the ones to develop the plant's full potential as a food source.

- Soy found its way to Europe at around 1500 A.D. Soy historian Dr. Theodore Hymowitz credits Benjamin Franklin with bringing soybean samples back to the United States from Paris's Jardin des Plantes. Whether or not this tale is true, by the early nineteenth century, soybeans were planted commercially in the United States.

- During the Civil War, soybeans were "brewed" as a coffee substitute. In 1904, George Washington Carver, who found many commercial uses for the peanut, began studying the soybean at the Tuskeegee Institute in Alabama.

- The United States produces half of the world's soybeans, making it the country's second biggest cash crop; there are 440,000 soybean farmers producing 2 billion bushels of soybeans a year. In fact, the United States exports much of its soybean crop to Japan and other Asian countries.

- In the 1970s, tofu became popular as an "environmentally friendly" food alternative to beef. People who were concerned about worldwide starvation and about conserving the earth's resources advocated tofu as a cheaper and more efficient source of protein than animal products. Popular books such as Frances Moore Lappe's *Diet for a Small Planet* and William Shurtleff and Akiko Aoyagi Shurtleff's *The Book of Tofu* promoted vegetarian, soy-based diets. Their argument was convincing: Beef cattle grazing on one acre of land can produce enough meat to sustain a person for seventy-seven days. If planted with soybeans, that same acre can produce enough protein to sustain a person for almost two and a half years. Indeed, many environmentally concerned people switched from meat to tofu, or at least cut down on meat consumption for the sake of the earth.

- Today many more people are switching to tofu and other soy products, not to save the world, but to save themselves from modern-day plagues such as cancer and heart disease. People are turning to soy foods out of concern for their health, and the marketplace is responding to these concerns.

- According to the Soyfoods Center, a group that tracks soy use worldwide, there are a record 500 new soy foods coming on the market each year, adding to the 12,000 soy foods already available.

Two

Soy by any Other Name

The soybean is a legume belonging to the genus *Glycine*. It is related to clover, peas, and alfalfa. There are two types of soybeans: *Glycine max* refers to the cultivated soybean; *Glycine soja* refers to the wild soybean. The edible portion—the soybean—actually is the seed from the soy pod. Young soybeans are found in green, fuzzy pods, but as they mature they turn brown and ripen into hard, dry beans.

Soybeans, or soy products, are sometimes referred to as *soya*. According to the *Soya Bluebook,* a leading trade reference, *soya* is a word used to describe the "plant, crop or category of products derived from soybeans."

Long before chemists were able to analyze foods down to the

nearest molecule, the Chinese called soy "the meat without bones," and the "cow of China." Even before people knew what protein was, the Chinese suspected that soybeans were a source of a nutrient that was essential for life.

Protein is necessary for building new tissues, transporting oxygen and nutrients in the blood, making antibodies to fight infection and repairing and replacing tissues as the body needs them. There are two types of food protein: complete protein and incomplete protein. A *complete protein* contains all of the eight essential amino acids that cannot be produced by the body: tryptophan, phenylalanine, lysine, threonine, methionine, leucine, isoleucine, and valine. (However, infants and small children require additional methionine in their diets.) Complete proteins are usually found in foods of animal origin such as eggs and meat. However, soy is one of the few plant foods that contain the proper balance of the eight essential amino acids. In particular, soy is abundant in lysine, an amino acid that is usually scarce in plant foods.

When foods can be combined to form complete proteins, they are called *complementing proteins*. As with other vegetable proteins, the nutritional value of soy is enhanced by eating it with a grain such as rice, pasta, or bread, which may offer different types of essential amino acids.

The U.S. government recognizes soy as a protein alternative equivalent to meat. In 1980, the U.S. Armed Forces began using soy extender in ground beef. In 1983, the U.S. Department of Agriculture (USDA) approved the use of soy protein as a partial substitute for meat products in school lunches and other programs. Soy-based infant formula is considered as good a protein source as milk-based formula and is given to full-term infants who are allergic to cow's milk. (Premature infants often require more protein than is found in either human milk or soy milk.) In fact, according to a recent article on soy products that appeared in the *American Journal of Clinical Nutrition,* "It can be concluded that, except for premature infants, soy protein can serve as a sole protein source in the human body."

Soy has several advantages over animal protein: It is low in fat as compared to most forms of meat, has no cholesterol, and is also a good source of isoflavones and other important phytochemicals that may protect against cancer and heart disease. Whole soybeans are a good source of fiber and minerals such as iron, calcium, phosphorus, magnesium, and the B vitamins thiamin, riboflavin, and niacin. However, with the exception of tempeh, a fermented soybean product popular in Indonesia, soybeans are a poor source of Vitamin B_{12}, a vitamin that is involved in red-blood-cell production and is found primarily in foods of animal origin. For that reason, vegetarians should take supplementary B_{12} (see Chapter 10).

Raw and unprocessed soybeans are tough and unappetizing. In addition, they contain compounds called *protease inhibitors* (also known as *trypsin inhibitors*) that may hamper the digestion of protein in the body. Routine heat processing deactivates most of the trypsin inhibitors. However, commercial soy protein products still contain up to 20 percent residual protease inhibitors, which is not believed to be significant enough to interfere with protein absorption. (Protease inhibitors are not all bad—in fact, studies show that they may be potent anticarcinogens that can block the formation of malignant growths.)

Unprocessed soybeans also contain another "antinutrient" —phytic acid—which may interfere with the absorption of minerals such as calcium and iron. Traditionally, soy processors have tried to rid the soybean of this "troublesome" compound, however recent studies suggest that its affect on mineral absorption may be minimal. In addition, phytic acid is being investigated as a potential cancer fighter.

Whole dried soybeans contain 40 percent protein and are a good source of fiber. Dried soybeans can be cooked like any other bean and used in casseroles, eaten as a side dish, or made into a vegetarian croquette or burger. However, in its purest form soybeans have a strong "beany" flavor that may not be to everyone's liking. Similar to other legumes, soybeans contain several sugars that human enzymes cannot digest. Although cooking reduces the amount of indigestible material, some people find that eating whole soybeans can cause flatulence. Dried, whole soybeans are sold in natural food stores.

Soy nuts, which are very popular in the West, are deep-fried or dry-roasted soybeans that are often salted or flavored with seasoning. They are also used as an ingredient in candy, cookies, and other baked goods. Soy nuts are an excellent source of protein, fiber, and isoflavones, however like true nuts they are high in fat and calories. Soy nuts are sold in natural food stores.

Soy sprouts are whole soybeans that have been sprouted for up to six days. Soy sprouts are terrific in stir-fried vegetable dishes, and are a good source of protein and fiber. Soy sprouts are sold in natural food stores and greengrocers.

Fresh green soybeans are the bean and pod. They can be steamed and eaten as a fresh vegetable; indeed, when cooked until tender, the fuzzy green pods are sweet and delicious. Unlike dried soybeans, fresh soybeans are eaten young. Soybean in the pod, known as *eda-mame,* is a popular snack in Japan and is served in many natural foods restaurants in the United States. If you've never tasted *eda-mame,* you're in for a treat! Green soybeans are a good source of protein, fiber, and isoflavones.

Traditional Soy Foods

For thousands of years soy has been a mainstay of traditional Asian cuisines. Many of the soy products in these cuisines have found their way to the United States and are rapidly growing in popularity.

Soy Milk

Soy milk is a creamy, milklike beverage that is made by soaking and grinding whole soybeans with water. It can also be made by adding water to whole, full-fat soy flour. Soy milk is lactose free and is often used by people who are lactose intolerant or allergic to cow's milk. Unfortified soy milk is packed with protein, B vitamins and minerals; it does not contain as much calcium, Vitamin D, or B_{12} as regular milk. However, some brands are fortified with Vitamin D, calcium, and B_{12}. Soy milk is a good source of isoflavones.

In Asian countries, fresh soy milk is sold by vendors on the street. Yuba, the skin that forms on the freshly made soy milk, is carefully saved and dried. It is then sold in flat sheets or in rolls and used as a confection or in cooking. Soy viili is a yogurtlike product that is made by adding a bacterial culture to soy milk.

Soy milk is sold in natural food stores and in many supermarkets in the United States. Soy milk sales in the United States have soared in recent years, largely owing to improved processing techniques that have virtually eliminated the undesirable "beany" flavor typical of early soy milk. Today, soy milk has a light, delicious flavor. It is sold plain or in a variety of flavors including chocolate, almond, malt, mocha, and vanilla. (Flavored soy milk may have a lower isoflavone content than plain.) Consumers have a choice of full-fat or low-fat soy milk. Many stores also sell dried soy milk. Soy milk is sold in aseptic 1-quart and 8-ounce containers that do not need refrigeration, as well as in refrigerated plastic 1-quart and half-gallon containers.

Soy milk can be drunk as a hot or cold beverage, poured over cold cereal, or used in cooking as a substitute for dairy products.

Tofu

Of all the soy foods, tofu is perhaps the most well known. Also called *bean curd,* tofu is a mild-tasting, white, cheeselike cake made from soy milk. Tofu comes in many different forms and can be used in an infinite number of ways. It is unique among

foods in that it can literally soak up any flavor that is added to
it. Tofu works equally well in a zesty chili as a meat substitute
for ground beef and in chocolate "cheese" cake as a substitute
for dairy cream cheese. Tofu can be used as a cheese substitute
in lasagna or can be barbecued on a grill. It is also delicious
diced into a bowl of miso soup or consommé with scallions
and fresh vegetables. This versatile food is high in protein,
relatively low in fat (it comes in both full-fat and low-fat varieties), is cholesterol-free, low in sodium, and an excellent
source of isoflavones.

No one knows precisely when tofu was invented, however it
is believed to be more than two thousand years old. According
to one Chinese legend, tofu was discovered by an honest government official during the Tang dynasty. Too poor to afford
meat because he refused to accept bribes, this official suppos-
edly created tofu out of desperation. Another legend attributes
the discovery of tofu to a Chinese alchemist, Prince Lord Liu An
of Huia-nam. Tofu was introduced in Japan in around 700 A.D.

Tofu is made from dried soybeans that are soaked in water
and then crushed and boiled. The remaining liquid, or soy
milk, is separated from the pulp or *okara,* which is also used as
a food. A coagulant (curdling agent) is added to the soy milk
to make it separate into curds and whey. The fresh, warm
curds are then poured into square molds, and several hours
later they become firm. Traditionally, tofu is stored in cool
water to keep it fresh. Several different coagulants may be used,
including nigari, a compound naturally occurring in seawater,
or calcium sulfate, a naturally occurring mineral. (Tofu made
with calcium sulfate is an excellent source of calcium.)

There are several different types of tofu:

- **Firm tofu** (also known as cotton tofu) has a solid consistency. During the tofu-making process, a cotton cloth is
  used to drain water from the curds, resulting in a denser
  product. Firm tofu is excellent in cooked dishes when you
  want the tofu to maintain its shape and consistency. It is
  higher in protein, fat, and calcium than other forms of tofu.

Some brands of tofu come in extra firm, which has a slightly denser consistency than firm.

- **Silken tofu,** or soft tofu, is tofu in which the water is not drained from the curds, leaving it with a softer, creamier consistency. Silken tofu is good pureed or blended.

- **Yakidofu** is tofu that has been lightly broiled and has a firm texture. It is often used in dishes such as sukiyaki (a one-pot dish including beef slices, tofu, and vegetables).

- **Koyodofu** is freeze-dried tofu that is sold in small, airtight packages and is especially good at soaking up the flavor of soups and broths. It is beige colored with a spongy texture. (Freeze-dried tofu must be reconstituted before using it in cooking.)

Okara, the soybean pulp that is separated from the soy milk during the tofu-making process, can also be used in cooking and is packed with protein and fiber. It is tasty in salads and soups or to make croquettes or even muffins. Okara is a heart-healthful food: recent animal studies show that okara is an excellent cholesterol-lowering agent.

Tofu is easily available almost everywhere in the United States. It is sold in supermarkets, greengrocers, Asian food shops, and natural food stores. Tofu is packaged in a variety of ways. Fresh tofu is often sold loose and is stored floating in basins of water.

Firm tofu may contain up to 6 grams of fat; silken tofu contains around 5 grams of fat. Although full-fat tofu is still relatively low in fat compared to meat, fat-gram counters take note: as of this writing, there are at least two brands of low-fat tofu on the market (see page 235). Powdered, instant tofu mix is also sold in many natural foods and Asian food stores. It is no more difficult to make than instant pudding, but it is somewhat more expensive than fresh tofu.

In Japan, there are more than 30,000 tofu shops that sell nothing but different varieties of tofu!

Natto

Natto is made from whole cooked soybeans that are fermented by adding a culture of *Bacillus natto* until the mixture develops a sticky coating. Natto has a cheeselike texture and a pungent smell, and is used in Japanese cooking in spreads or in soups. Natto is a good source of protein and isoflavones. Since it includes the whole soybean, it is also high in fiber.

Tempeh

Tempeh is a fermented soybean patty made from whole soybeans that are soaked overnight and then briefly cooked until they are softened. A dry powder of the mold *Rhizopus oryzae* (a tempeh starter) is added to the cooked soybeans and the mixture is allowed to stand for twenty-four hours. The final product has a slightly nutty, mildly smoky flavor that is similar to mushrooms and a chewy, meatlike texture. Tempeh can be grilled, fried, or grated and made into into vegetarian burgers, or diced as a chicken substitute in mock chicken salad.

Tempeh, which dates back more than two thousand years, is an Indonesian specialty. In fact, in Indonesia, street vendors sell tempeh on the street, wrapped in banana leaves or on a skewer, seasoned with satay sauce. Tempeh is fast becoming popular in the West, and is featured on the menus of many natural food restaurants and can be found in most natural foods stores.

Tempeh is usually sold in 6- or 8-ounce packages, and is often frozen. Be sure to buy the freshest product available. Fresh tempeh can keep in the refrigerator for about ten days; frozen tempeh can last in the freezer for several months. Similar to other fermented or aged products, mold may form on tempeh. Fresh tempeh will have white flecks; stale tempeh will have black flecks and may have a bitter flavor.

Tempeh is rich in protein, fiber, vitamins, minerals, and isoflavones. Unlike most other soy products, it is also a good source of vitamin B_{12}, which is a by-product of the fermentation process and usually found only in foods of animal origin. (The B_{12} content may vary from batch to batch.)

Miso

Miso is a fermented bean paste made by mixing soybeans, salt, and water with *koji,* a cultured grain (usually rice or barley) used as a starter. The culture is then aged in cedar vats for up to three years. Miso has a distinctive, robust flavor. It is packed with protein and isoflavones, low in fat, but high in sodium. Therefore, it should not be eaten by people who are sodium sensitive or who have high blood pressure, and should be used sparingly by everyone else.

Miso is very versatile. It can be used as a condiment, made into a soup, and even used as a base for salad dressing or barbecue sauce. Most Japanese eat several spoonfuls of miso daily. Millions of Japanese start their day with a hot bowl of miso soup. There are several types of miso, which vary according to color and taste. Light, or yellow miso is sweet and less salty than darker miso and is often used in salad dressings. Red miso (made with barley) makes a terrific stock for vegetable soup. The darker miso tends to be stronger and denser than the lighter varieties and also makes a hearty base for soup.

In the United States, miso can be found at natural food stores and Asian food stores. Asian markets are packed with different types of miso: real aficionados can distinguish between brands, which may vary according to processing techniques. The "quick" misos, which are produced with little or no time to age, are usually not as good as misos made in the classical Asian style. Miso can be stored in the refrigerator for up to a year.

Studies have shown that miso may help rid the body of radioactive elements. According to the Japanese Economic Newswire, Dr. Shinichiro Akizuki, of Saint Francis Hospital in Nagasaki, observed that physicians who came to Nagaski to

treat atomic bomb victims in 1945, after the bomb was
dropped, did not suffer from radiation poisoning. In his book,
Food and Predispositions, Dr. Akizuki theorized that compounds
in miso soup and seaweed may have protected the physicians
from the harmful effects of the residual radiation. Dr. Akizuki's
book was sold in Europe; after the Soviet nuclear reactor ac-
cident at Chernobyl, European orders for Japanese miso sky-
rocketed.

Soy Sauce

Soy sauce, known as *shoyu,* may be the most popular condiment in the world. It is widely used as a seasoning in Asian
cooking, and has also found its way into Western cuisine. Soy
sauce is made by adding spores from an *Aspergillus* mold to a
mixture of roasted soybeans and wheat. The culture (called
koji) is grown for three days and then mixed with saltwater and
brewed in fermentation tanks for up to one year. The liquid
from the resulting product is further refined and pasteurized.
Chinese soy sauce has a strong flavor and is very salty. Japanese
soy sauce is somewhat lighter and sweeter. Light soy sauce is
lighter in color, thinner, and saltier than dark soy sauce. Tamari, which is sold in natural food stores, is similar to soy sauce
in taste and is often used as a basting sauce.

Dutch traders brought soy sauce back to Europe in the
seventh century. According to *Japanese Cooking: A Simple Art*
by Shizuo Tsuji, soy sauce was the secret seasoning used at the
court banquets of Louis XIV of France.

In the United States, soy sauce is sold in supermarkets, Asian
markets, and natural food stores. Naturally fermented soy
sauce is superior in quality and taste to synthetic soy sauce. Be
sure to buy only naturally brewed soy sauce! Soy sauce is very
salty, and should not be consumed by people who are salt
sensitive or who have high blood pressure. Low-sodium soy
sauce, which is sold in many supermarkets, is preferable to
regular soy sauce.

Soy does not contain isoflavones, however some studies suggest that it may have other anticarcinogenic compounds. In fact, according to one study published in *Cancer Research,* researchers at the University of Wisconsin tested the effect of soy sauce on laboratory mice who had been fed a carcinogen known for inducing stomach cancer. The rats who had been given soy sauce along with their daily food had significantly fewer tumors than those who had not.

Kinnoko Flour

In Japan, roasted soybeans are ground to a fine powder that is then used to make sweets. Kinnoko is a good source of protein and isoflavones. Products made with kinnoko can be found at Asian markets in the United States.

Soy Protein Products

In the United States, 90 percent of all soy products are consumed in the form of soy protein. Typically, soybeans are processed to create these food products and ingredients. In processing, the soybeans are dried to eliminate excess moisture and are then cracked, dehulled, and rolled into flakes. The soy hulls are an excellent source of fiber. Oil is extracted from the soybeans, and the defatted soy flakes are processed into various soy protein products.

Soy Protein Concentrates

Soy concentrate is at least 65 percent protein, dry weight. This product is often used as a meat extender or to give a protein boost to commercially prepared products, or to improve texture or the "mouth feel" in products such as frozen TV dinners. By itself, soy protein concentrate has a discernible soy flavor and is rarely used by consumers in cooking.

Soy Protein Isolate

Soy protein isolate, or isolated soy protein, is sold in the form of a powder (either plain or flavored) that contains at least 90 percent protein. It is fat-free and carbohydrate-free and is a fair source of isoflavones. Soy protein isolate is highly versatile and can be used in a variety of ways, as in a meat extender to reduce the fat and cholesterol content of foods such as burgers. It is also used as a milk replacement in nondairy creamers. Because it is a nonfat source of high-quality protein, soy protein isolate is commonly used in powdered weight-loss beverages. It can also be found in meal-replacement bars, infant formula, and "muscle-building" protein powders.

Recent studies show that soy protein isolate can be a potent cholesterol-lowering agent. According to several studies, substituting soy protein for some animal protein can yield a substantial reduction in blood-cholesterol levels over a relatively short time (see "Lowering Your Cholesterol with Soy," page 63). As a result, there has been growing consumer interest in this product. Isolated soy protein can be used in baking or cooking, or it can be sprinkled on cereal or even blended with juice or fruit for a nondairy shake.

Soy protein isolate, either flavored or plain, can be purchased at many natural food stores under many different labels. General Nutrition Center sells a product that is 95 percent pure isolated soy protein. Twin Labs (under the name of Veggie Fuel) and Fearns (a division of Modern Products) also market forms of isolated soy protein. Soy protein drinks (such as Nature's Plus Spiru-tein) are also easy to find in most natural food stores. Don't confuse soy protein isolate with products labeled "soy protein." In some cases, "soy protein" could refer to soy flour, which is lower in protein than isolated soy protein and often higher in fat. If you can't find plain soy protein isolate in your area, look for a protein powder in which soy protein isolate is listed as the first or second ingredient. (For more information on where to buy soy protein isolate, see page 237.)

Soy Flour

The "meat" from the roasted soybean is rolled into flakes and then finely ground into a powder that can be used in baking. It contains no less than 50 percent protein and is an excellent source of isoflavones. Soy flour is widely used in commercial baking, and is becoming popular for home baking, especially among vegetarians who want to add a protein boost to their home-baked goods. Soy flour can also add moisture and a delicate nutty flavor to food.

Full-fat soy flour can be very high in fat; look for defatted or "low-fat" soy flour, in which the oil has been extracted from the flakes during processing. Defatted soy flour is also a more concentrated source of protein. Soy flour is gluten-free, however, and so cannot be used as a substitute for wheat or rye flour in yeast-raised breads. In products not yeast raised, you can substitute about 20 percent of the total flour with soy flour. Soy flour is heavier than other flours; if you use too much, it can result in a product that is too dense.

Soy flour may help prevent fat absorption during the frying process. Studies have shown that doughnuts made with soy flour absorbed significantly less fat during deep-frying than doughnuts made with other types of flour. Soy flour is also good for microwave baking since it helps retain moisture. Soy flour is sold in natural food stores.

Texturized Soy Protein

When is a meatloaf not a meatloaf? When it's made from the "meat" of the soybean. Texturized soy protein (TSP) is made from soy flour that is compressed until the protein fibers change in structure. TSP is high in protein, isoflavones, calcium, iron, and zinc and low in fat and calories. When dry, TSP has a texture similar to granola. TSP must be rehydrated before it can be used in recipes. It can be used to replace part or all of the ground beef in dishes such as chili, meatloaf, or hamburgers. TSP is sold in natural food stores and some supermarkets.

Meat Analogs

Soy protein can be made into a variety of nonmeat foods that look, smell, and practically taste like the real thing. Soy-based cold cuts, imitation bacon and sausage, and vegetarian hamburger, chili, and hot dogs are available at natural food stores and in most supermarkets. They are sold as frozen, canned, or dried foods. Soy-based meat products are a good source of protein and are usually lower in fat and cholesterol than real meat. However, they are a poor source of isoflavones and unless they are vitamin fortified, will not have the same vitamin B_{12} content as animal foods. In addition, in some cases they are filled with chemical additives such as food dyes and preservatives which should be avoided.

Other Soy Products

Soy Fiber

Fiber is the portion of plant foods that is not digested in the gastrointestinal tract, but may be fermented by microflora in the large bowel. Soybeans, like other legumes, are a good source of fiber. One cup of cooked soybeans contain about 6 grams of fiber. During processing, soy fiber is derived from the dehulled, defatted soybean cotyledon (seed). Soy fiber is used in commercial liquid diets, in baked goods, and as a fiber supplement.

Soy fiber offers many potential health benefits. It speeds up the transit time of food through the intestine, which helps not only to prevent constipation but to ward off colon cancer. In animal and human studies, soy fiber lowered cholesterol in subjects with high cholesterol who also followed a low-fat, low-cholesterol diet. In other studies, soy fiber helped to stabilize blood glucose levels in diabetic patients.

Soybean Oil

Soy is the most widely used vegetable oil in the United States. It has a bland, light flavor that makes it suitable for cooking. Soy oil is a common ingredient in commercial baked goods, prepared foods, and salad dressings. Crude soybean oil is derived from edible, defatted soy flakes during processing; the oil is further refined before it is used as cooking oil. Although soy oil does not contain isoflavones, it does contain other beneficial compounds. Unlike most other vegetable oils, soy oil is rich in omega-3 and omega-6 fatty acids similar to those found in marine fish oils. Studies have shown that marine fish oils can cut blood cholesterol and triglyceride levels, lower blood pressure, and prevent blood clots. Soybean oil also contains linoleic acid, which is essential for life but cannot be produced by the body. Some studies suggest that linoleic acid may help prevent certain forms of cancer, including breast cancer and colorectal cancer. However, all oils should be used sparingly. Some studies show that a high amount of polyunsaturated fats can actually promote the growth of tumors.

Soy oil has a high smoking point that makes it good for sautéing or wok cooking, which require high heat. Like other oils, soy oil is calorie dense, weighing in at 9 calories per gram (as compared to protein and carbohydrate, which are 4 calories per gram).

As a rule of thumb, eat no more than 20 percent of your daily calories in the form of fat.

Lecithin

Lecithin is a by-product of soy oil. It is a natural emulsifier and lubricant, widely used in products ranging from candy bars to margarine to pharmaceuticals. Recently, lecithin has gained popularity among health-conscious consumers because of its reputation as a cholesterol-lowering agent. Lecithin can be purchased in capsule or granule form at natural food stores.

Questions about Soy Foods

I know that soy milk is often given to infants who are allergic to cow's milk. Is soy hypoallergenic?

Soy is not hypoallergenic. Although soy milk is usually given to infants who are allergic to cow's-milk protein, about 25 percent of babies allergic to cow's milk will also be allergic to the protein in soy milk. However, soy protein is less allergenic than milk protein and may cause fewer adverse reactions. Although food protein allergies primarily affect small children, there have been cases, albeit rare, of adults developing allergies to soy.

If the phytochemicals in soybeans are so healthy, why can't they be extracted from food and made into a pill like a vitamin?

There are many potentially beneficial phytochemicals in soy, including isoflavones, protease inhibitors, and phytic acid. Researchers are not certain which phytochemicals are the most important, and whether or not individual compounds work better combined with others or even with other phytochemicals. There may even be other beneficial compounds in soy that have yet to be identified. Your best bet is to eat the real food.

Many of the soy products sold in my local natural foods store are labeled "organically grown." Are organically grown soybeans better?

"Organic" means that a food is grown and shipped without the use of chemical pesticides, fungicides, synthetic fertilizers, waxes, or other chemical additives. Food that is labeled "organically grown" must comply with the National Organic Standards Law, which took effect in 1993. Under the act, organic farms must be monitored by state inspectors to make sure that the farming or processing procedures comply with guidelines. Many people prefer using organically grown produce because they do not want to ingest chemicals. They may also feel that organic farming practices are better for the environment. I personally opt for organic produce whenever I can get it. However, in the case of soybeans, even if the crop is sprayed, there is limited consumer exposure to any chemicals, since the beans are encased in a pod. Therefore, I think that most soy products on the market are reasonably safe, whether or not they have the organic label.

More Soy Miracles

The soyplant has been dubbed the "miracle crop" because of the numerous products that are spawned from its simple bean. Not only is soy a dietary staple for hundreds of millions of people worldwide but soy-based products are being used by industry as an environmentally friendly solution to some serious problems. Here are some examples of how soybeans help make the earth a healthier place.

- **Soy ink**—Chances are, your local newspaper is printed with soy ink, which is similar to regular ink except that soy oil replaces petroleum oil as a carrier for the pigment. Some of the largest printing plants in the country have made the switch from petroleum-based ink to soy ink, including the federal government, for several reasons. First, soy oil is better for the environment: during the manufacturing process it emits far less harmful fumes than petroleum, it's easier to remove from paper for recycling, and it helps conserve fossil fuel. Second, soy ink pleases readers because it looks good, but it doesn't rub off onto your fingers as easily as does petroleum ink.

- **Soy diesel**—In 1990, Congress passed the Clean Air Act, which mandated the use of cleaner-burning alternative fuels. Soy-based biodiesel fits the bill: it is a nontoxic, biodegradable, nonpolluting energy alternative. Soy-diesel blends reduce the amount of carbon monoxide and hydrocarbons produced when burned and lowers sulfur dioxide emissions from diesel engines. The fuel is manufactured in Kansas and Missouri, and is being used to run over a hundred diesel maintenance vehicles at St. Louis's Lambert Airport. Although soy diesel is currently too expensive to use on a widespread basis, researchers are investigating ways to make it more economically viable.

- **Soy plastics**—Researchers are exploring the use of soybean protein for a plastic that is easily biodegradable for short-term use, such as commercial food containers or plastic "throwaway" cutlery. The United States uses about 65 million pounds of plastic annually, and most is not recycled, which means it can linger in landfills for hundreds of years. Even if the plastic is recycled, second-hand plastics are not considered food-grade quality for use in packaging. Scientists hope to develop a soy plastic that is safe to use for food but that is also kind to the environment. Potentially, a soy protein container might even be ground up and used as animal feed!

- **Soy silk**—Researchers at the Georgia Institute of Technology in Atlanta are looking to put silkworms out of business. They are exploring the potential use of a soy-based silklike fabric that is both washable and relatively inexpensive.

- **Soy-based wood adhesives**—Researchers are investigating the possibility of a soy-based, nontoxic wood adhesive that could eliminate or substantially cut the emissions problems associated with formaldehyde-based adhesives. That's better for the environment and better for our lungs!

Soy's Top Ten Benefits

1. **Antioxidant.** Soy foods contain antioxidants— compounds which protect cells from damage caused by unstable oxygen molecules called *free radicals*. Free radicals are believed to be responsible for initiating many forms of cancer as well as premature aging. In addition, oxidation of LDL, or "bad cholesterol" is believed to promote the formation of plaque.

2. **Breast cancer.** A major study in Singapore revealed that women who eat soy foods are at lower risk of developing breast cancer than those who don't. Asian women, who typically eat a soy-based diet, have much lower levels of breast cancer than Western women. Test tube studies and those involving laboratory animals have shown that compounds in soy can inhibit the growth of breast cancer cells.

3. Cholesterol lowering. Scores of studies from around the world attest to soy's cholesterol-lowering properties, especially for people with high cholesterol levels.

4. Colon cancer. A recent U.S. study showed that Americans who made soybeans and tofu a regular part of their diet had significantly lower rates of colon cancer than those who didn't eat soy.

5. Hip fractures. Hip fractures owing to osteoporosis are a major problem among elderly women in the United States. Japanese women have half the rate of hip fractures as U.S. women; preliminary studies suggest that soy may help retain bone mass.

6. Hot flashes. Half of all menopausal women in the United States complain of hot flashes, a problem that is so rare in Japan that there's not even a word for it. Some researchers believe that special compounds in soy called *phytoestrogens* may help Japanese women stay cooler.

7. Immunity. Studies show that soybean peptides (chains of amino acids) can boost the immune system, helping the body to fight disease.

8. Kidney disease. Soy protein is easier on the kidneys, the main filtering organ of the body, than is animal protein and may slow down or prevent kidney damage in people with impaired kidney function.

9. Lung cancer. Studies have linked soy consumption to lower rates of lung cancer.

10. Prostate cancer. A major study of Japanese men in Hawaii found a direct correlation between consumption of tofu and lower rates of prostate cancer. Studies of soy compounds have shown that they can inhibit the growth of prostate cancer cells in laboratory cultures.

Three

Does Soy
Prevent Cancer?

According to the World Health Organization's chart of
cancer mortality rates for fifty countries, if you live in
the United States or just about any other industrialized
Western nation, your risk of dying from most types of cancer
is significantly higher than if you lived in one of several Asian
countries, including China, Japan, Republic of Korea, and Thai-
land. What is particularly striking is the comparatively high
mortality rates for breast cancer and prostate cancer in the
West. In fact, depending on which Western country you lived
in, your risk of dying of breast cancer or prostate cancer could
be as much as ten to twenty times greater than if you lived in
Asia!

Why is the death rate from certain types of cancers so much lower in Asia than in the West? Do Asians have special protection against these diseases? Although we don't know what causes cancer, we do know that, in most cases, genetics is only one small risk factor. That is, only a small number of these cancers can be attributed to heredity, which means that it is unlikely that any one race has "special protection." In addition, when Asians emigrate to Western countries, within one or two generations their descendants run the same risk of dying of cancer as do longer-term residents. In fact, in recent years, as the traditional Asian diet has become more Westernized, Asians have experienced a steady rise in mortality from breast and other types of cancer.

Most researchers agree that cancer is caused by the interplay of many different factors, including lifestyle, lifetime exposure to carcinogens (cancer-causing substances), and diet. Many studies have shown that people who eat a typical Western diet that is high in fat and low in fiber—just the opposite of the traditional Asian diet—are more prone to develop certain forms of cancer, especially hormone-dependent cancers such as prostate and breast cancers. These cancers are called hormone dependent because hormones can stimulate their growth.

As important as dietary fat and fiber may be as risk factors, cancer researchers are beginning to believe that which foods we eat may prove to be a major player in promoting or preventing cancer. Soybeans, a dietary staple in many Asian nations, contain many potentially beneficial compounds that may help prevent certain types of cancer. Several compounds in soy have generated great interest in the medical community, including:

- **Isoflavones**—These compounds are converted in the body into phytoestrogens (which literally means "plant estrogens"), hormonelike compounds that may help prevent the growth of hormone-dependent cancers.

- **Genistein**—Soy is the only source of genistein, an isoflavone that is receiving a great deal of attention from scientists. Laboratory experiments demonstrate that genistein can inhibit enzymes that promote tumor growth. Test tube and animal experiments have also shown that genistein can block the growth of prostate cancer cells and breast cancer cells. In addition, genistein can help promote a process called *differentiation* in cancerous cells. The human body is filled with specialized cells, such as bone cells, skin cells, and heart cells, that have unique properties. However, when cells become cancerous, they lose their former identity—that is, they "forget" what they were designed to do and begin to look the same. Undifferentiated cells are particularly resistant to cancer therapy.

- **Daidzein**—This is another isoflavone found in soy. Recent studies show that this compound can inhibit the growth of cancer cells and promote cell differentiation in animals.

- **Protease inhibitors**—These compounds block the action of proteases, enzymes that may promote tumor growth. According to Ann R. Kennedy, Ph.D., a leading researcher at the University of Pennsylvania School of Medicine, protease inhibitors may be a "universal anticarcinogen" that work in many different animals to prevent or inhibit a wide range of cancers, from liver cancer to colon cancer to breast cancer.

- **Phytic acid**—This compound is an antioxidant that is found in many plants. Phytic acid is a chelator—that is, it binds with certain metals that may promote tumor growth. Animal studies have shown that phytic acid can reduce the size and number of tumors in laboratory animals that were fed a potent carcinogen.

- **Saponins**—These compounds, which are found in soybeans, chickpeas, ginseng and sunflower seeds, have been shown in animal studies to kill colon-cancer cells.

In addition, several population studies have linked consumption of soy foods to a lower risk of certain cancers, including cancers of the breast, prostate, stomach, and lung. In fact, one study of men of Japanese ancestry living in Hawaii showed that eating tofu was the single factor that appeared to lower their risk of developing prostate cancer. In another study performed in Singapore, researchers compared the diets of 200 Chinese women with breast cancer to the diets of 420 cancer-free women. They found a strong correlation between consumption of soy foods and a decreased risk of developing breast cancer.

Although researchers aren't certain why soy may prevent cancer—or which compounds in soy may be the most effective—they do have some interesting theories. This chapter examines the different ways soy may protect you against various types of cancer.

Phytoestrogens: They May Look Like Hormones But . . .

Phytoestrogens and their potential ability to prevent cancer are two of the hottest areas in scientific research today. Phytoestrogens are plant compounds that are converted during the normal digestive process into a form of very weak estrogen. Soybeans are particularly rich in phytoestrogens. Although phytoestrogens may be thousands of times weaker than the steroidal hormones naturally produced by the body, these plant derived compounds can still exert a powerful influence.

For example, in 1946, a mysterious outbreak of infertility among Australian sheep nearly decimated the sheep industry in Southwest Australia, until it was discovered that the clover the ewes grazed on was especially rich in phytoestrogens. These plant hormones altered the ewes' normal hormonal balance, resulting in sterility.

No one suspected that phytoestrogens could have an affect on humans until several decades later. In 1982, Kenneth Setchell, Ph.D., now professor of pediatrics at Children's Hospital and Medical Center in Cincinnati, identified a new phytoestrogen, equol, in the urine of people who eat soy foods. Equol was of particular interest to researchers because of its structural similarity to the natural estrogen, estradiol-17. In a later study, Dr. Herman Adlercreutz of the University of Helsinki found high levels of equol in the urine of Japanese men and women consuming the traditional Asian diet, notably rich in soy. In other studies, Dr. Adlercreutz found low levels of equol in women with breast cancer, as opposed to cancer-free women. In order to understand the importance of these discoveries, it's necessary to grasp the role of hormones in the human body, and how phytoestrogens—and soy—may alter that role.

Reigning Hormones

When a teenager begins to misbehave, we often attribute his or her behavior to "raging hormones." But it's not just teenagers who are controlled by hormones. At any age, hormones are involved in nearly all our bodily functions. Hormones are sometimes called chemical messengers because they carry messages to cells all over the body, influencing activities such as growth, metabolism, and sexual development. The hormone estrogen is also involved in many other activities, including cholesterol transport and bone building. In women, estrogen controls the development of secondary sexual characteristics such as breasts. In men, the hormone testosterone controls secondary characteristics such as facial hair and muscle growth. Both men and women produce estrogen and testosterone, however women produce more estrogen and men produce more testosterone.

Estrogen is a major player in the female menstrual cycle. In a delicate interplay with other hormones, estrogen stimulates the development of the ovum (unfertilized egg) and helps to grow the lining of the uterus, where the egg will implant if it is fertilized.

A woman's level of available estrogen is regulated by a complex feedback mechanism. Only 1 to 2 percent of the estrogen in the body circulates freely in the bloodstream; the rest is bound to another protein. Bound estrogen is inactive—that is, it does not exert an influence on other tissues and cannot promote cell growth. But as the body needs estrogen, an enzyme frees it so it can circulate through the body. When the circulating estrogen level gets too low, more of the bound estrogen is released into the bloodstream. When estrogen levels rise too high, less is released.

Free estrogen, called *estradiol,* is a more potent form of the hormone that is sent to targeted organs. It binds to cells with special estrogen receptors—so-called estrogen-sensitive cells. Once bound, the estrogen triggers a chain of reactions that can influence cell behavior, sometimes in detrimental ways.

The Cancer Connection

A healthy cell knows precisely how to grow, when to divide, and when to stop—this is called the *cell cycle.* But if the genetic information in the cell—its DNA—is injured or altered, the cell may begin to behave erratically. The term *cancer* describes many different diseases in which cells begin to grow out of control and form masses called *tumors,* which can turn malignant and spread throughout the body.

What causes a healthy cell to go awry? No one knows precisely why some cells begin to grow wildly out of control, however many researchers believe that the onset of cancer occurs in two phases; with an initiator and a promoter.

The first phase involves an initiator—the substance that actually inflicts the initial damage to the cell causing it to mutate. Many cancer researchers suspect that the initiators of different types of cancers are free radicals (unstable oxygen molecules), which can attack cell membranes and alter the DNA. Ultraviolet light, tobacco, heavy metals, chemicals, lipids, alcohol, and radiation all are substances that can promote the formation of free radicals. In some cases, a virus may also be an initiator.

Those mutated cells can lay dormant for years. In the second phase of the cancer process, a promoter or proliferator "awakens" these cells and encourages them to start dividing, thus the tumor begins to multiply and spread. For more than a century, scientists have recognized that estrogen may be a cancer promoter. In the 1880s, doctors observed that tumors shrunk in women with breast cancer who underwent removal of their ovaries, the body's major producer of estrogen. In 1948, several hundred women with breast cancer who had undergone radical mastectomies also underwent radiation to their ovaries, which put them into an early menopause. The women who had the radiation lived longer than women who had just had mastectomies. Since then, hormonal therapy involving manipulation of hormone levels has been an important treatment for breast cancer and other hormone-dependent cancers.

Although researchers acknowledge a connection between estrogen and cancer, the exact mechanism is unknown. The most common belief is that when estrogen binds to a receptor site on an already altered cell, it stimulates the cell to grow and divide in abnormal ways. Many studies have shown that when a cell is exposed to estrogen, it speeds up the cell cycle—that is, it interferes with the cell's normal, orderly mechanism for regulating its growth. Estrogen receptor sites have been found on cancers in the breast, prostate, and endometrium (uterine lining) and even in the colon and thyroid.

Lifetime exposure to potent forms of estrogen may be a risk factor for hormone-dependent cancers. Some studies suggest that the risk of breast cancer increases among women who begin to menstruate early and have a late menopause, presumably because they have been exposed to potent estrogens for a longer period. Remaining childless is another risk factor for breast cancer, since during pregnancy there are less active forms of circulating estrogen than during menstruation.

Even though estrogen levels drop after menopause, menopausal women are at a much higher risk of developing breast cancer. Weight gain, which often accompanies aging, may be a contributing factor. In postmenopausal women, some hormones are converted into estrogen by fat cells; thus, the greater the number of fat cells, the greater the output of estrogen.

In men, estrogen works somewhat differently but it can be equally destructive. Estrogen is a precursor to androgens, or male hormones—that is, it can trigger the production of testosterone by signaling the brain to produce another hormone that, in turn, stimulates the testes to produce more testosterone. Studies have shown that men with prostate cancer often have higher levels of active testosterone than men who are cancer free.

Fooling Mother Nature

Many researchers believe that phytoestrogens may help manipulate the hormonal environment in a favorable way, and by doing so, may help prevent hormone-dependent cancers from developing. Phytoestrogens are structurally similar to the estrogen that is produced by the body—so similar, in fact, that they can literally fool cells into thinking they are the real thing. Although these phytoestrogens are far weaker than natural estrogen, if they occur in high enough concentrations they can "outcompete" the natural estrogens for binding spots on estrogen-sensitive cells. The theory goes that if the estrogen receptor sites are already occupied by the weaker phytoestrogens, the more potent forms of estrogen cannot bind, and are prevented from causing destructive changes in the cells.

Several studies have shown that women with a high amount of phytoestrogens have lower levels of potent estrogens than women who do not. For example, one recent study compared estrogen levels among Japanese women to those of American Caucasian women. The researchers chose to study Japanese women living in rural areas to ensure that they were eating the traditional Japanese diet, which is lower in fat and higher in soy products (a rich source of phytoestrogens) than the diet of women living in industrialized cities. Even after adjustment for their increased weight and larger body size, the estrogen levels in American women were significantly higher than those of the Japanese women. The researchers noted that the higher estrogen levels could explain why American women are four times more likely to die from breast cancer than Japanese women.

Phytoestrogens and the Menstrual Cycle

Phytoestrogens may alter the menstrual cycle in a way that may reduce the risk of developing breast cancer. In a study performed by Dr. Kenneth Setchell, premenopausal women with a history of regular menstrual cycles were given 60 grams of soy protein (slightly more than 2 ounces) for one month, then taken off the protein for another month, and then given the soy protein again for a third month. During the soy protein regime, the length of the menstrual cycle was extended by up to five days. More important, the follicular stage, or first half of the cycle, was increased and the luteal phase, or second half, was decreased. Breast cell division is greatest during the luteal phase, which may trigger the growth of latent tumors. In addition, Dr. Setchell speculates that women who eat soy may have fewer menstrual cycles over their lifetime, thus reducing their lifetime exposure to potent estrogen.

All About Genistein

Soy's ability to create a favorable hormonal environment is just one explanation for how this food may help prevent cancer. However, some researchers believe that soy's protective effect is due primarily to the action of one compound that can be found only in soy—genistein.

In November 1993, an article by Dr. Herman Adlercreutz published in the British medical journal *Lancet* attracted attention among both the lay and the medical community. It suggested that genistein may protect against prostate cancer. The article was cited in the *Wall Street Journal,* and it was the first time most people (including many physicians) had even heard of genistein.

Genistein was identified as a plant estrogen in 1966. However, it took more than two decades for genistein to be "discovered" by the medical community after a team of Japanese researchers found it had anticancer attributes. The researchers were looking for compounds that could stop the epidermal growth factor (EGF)—the enzyme which regulates cell growth and division—from becoming activated. The team found that genistein, an isoflavone unique to soy, was a "specific inhibitor for tyrosine kinase," which meant that it blocked the enzymes that lead to the activation of EGF. They speculated that "a specific inhibitor for tyrosine kinases could be an antitumor agent. . . ." In other words, anything that could block the signal that triggered cells to grow could also inhibit the growth of cancer.

Suddenly, genistein became a hot commodity as other researchers began to investigate its potential as a cancer protector. Most agree that genistein holds great promise as a way to prevent certain forms of cancer, and some even believe that it may one day be used as a possible cancer treatment.

Several studies have examined genistein's role as a cancer fighter. Autopsies of Japanese men show that prostate cancer is as common in Japan as it is in the United States, but the cancer seems to grow much more slowly—so slowly in fact, that many men die without ever developing clinical disease. Until recently, there was no explanation for this phenomenon. However, researchers now suspect that genistein is blocking the growth of these tumors. Finnish researcher Herman Adlercreutz and colleagues compared blood plasma levels of isoflavones in Japanese and Finnish men. The levels of isoflavones were more than one hundred times higher among the Japanese men, with genistein occurring in the highest concentration of any other isoflavone. The researchers concluded, "A life-long high concentration of isoflavonoids in plasma (Japanese children have as high a urinary excretion as adults) might explain why Japanese men have small latent carcinomas that seldom develop to clinical disease" (Lancet, November 13, 1993).

An international group of researchers headed by Theodore Fotsis of Children's University Hospital in Heidelberg found yet another potential mechanism by which genistein can prevent the spread of cancer. Angiogenesis is the generation of new capillaries or small blood vessels. Under normal circumstances, angiogenesis is a tightly controlled process that can occur only under certain conditions, including wound healing and during pregnancy to support the placenta. However, the presence of a tumor can induce angiogenesis: the tumor needs the new capillaries to deliver nourishment so it can grow. In this study, genistein was shown to block the process of angiogenesis in laboratory studies. It's possible that genistein may do the same thing in humans, however more studies need to be done.

Researchers Greg Peterson and Stephen Barnes of the University of Alabama tested whether genistein could block the growth of non-estrogen-dependent human breast-cancer cells. In this study, they showed that genistein thwarted the growth of breast cancer in vitro, and that the presence of an estrogen receptor is not necessary for isoflavones to inhibit tumor growth. This suggests that the protective effect of isoflavones may not be due to their effect on hormones but, rather, the particular ability of genistein to block cell growth.

Genistein holds great promise as a potential cancer protector. However, more studies need to be done to confirm whether genistein is a true cancer protector.

Phytic Acid

Why do the seeds of some plants remain viable for up to 400 years? Researchers speculate that phytic acid—a major ingredient in grains, nuts, legumes (including soybeans), and oil seeds—may play a role in extending the longevity of seeds. Many researchers also believe that phytic acid may help keep people healthy.

Phytic acid is an antioxidant—that is, it protects seeds against oxidative damage from free radicals or unstable oxygen molecules, which can cause mutations in DNA. Phytic acid's antioxidant activity is due to the fact that it is a chelator, which means that it binds easily to metal. In fact, phytic acid has a strong affinity for iron: it will search out and bind to iron before binding with other metals. In the presence of oxygen, iron can create free radicals that attack DNA. Phytic acid can prevent this damage from occurring by binding with the iron, thus keeping it away from oxygen.

Phytic acid not only protects seeds from oxidative damage but may well offer the same benefit to people who eat the food that is grown from the seeds. In several animal studies, phytic acid has been shown to inhibit the growth of tumors, especially in the colon. However, phytic acid appears in food that tends to be high in fiber, and fiber intake has also been linked to lower rates of colon and other forms of cancer. Some scientists speculate that it is the phytic acid, not the fiber, that actually protects against certain forms of cancer. In fact, in one review of phytic acid published in *Free Radical Biology and Medicine* (Vol. 8, 1990), researchers noted that in populations where people eat high quantities of red meat, which is rich in iron, "the simultaneous presence of phytate may act to suppress iron-driven steps in carcinogenesis."

The fiber–phytic acid debate is bound to go on for some time. However, everyone agrees that both are important, and Americans don't get enough of either one. Ironically, until recently, phytic acid was considered unhealthy because it inhibited the absorption of minerals. However, new research suggests that it may be just what the doctor ordered!

Protease Inhibitors

Protease inhibitors are compounds that inhibit the action of certain enzymes that promote tumor growth. At one time, protease inhibitors were considered carcinogenic. Early studies suggested that the protease inhibitors in raw soybeans could cause pancreatic cancer in rats, and soy processors quickly developed ways to remove them from soybeans. During heat processing, the level of protease inhibitors in soy products is greatly reduced, however it is not eliminated.

Some researchers contend that, even at this low level, protease inhibitors are powerful anticarcinogens. They also believe that the protease inhibitors are not responsible for triggering pancreatic cancer in rats; rather, the cancer is due to fat in the whole soybean. (Fat has been shown to promote tumor growth.) Other researchers point out that the kind of pancreatic cancer found in rats who eat raw soybeans is very rare in humans. They also note that in populations where large amounts of soy are consumed, the rate of pancreatic cancer is lower than in countries where little soy is eaten.

Soy contains a unique protease inhibitor—the Bowman-Birk Inhibitor (BBI)—that, according to researcher Dr. Ann Kennedy of the University of Pennsylvania School of Medicine, may prove to be a potent anticarcinogen. In a medical paper, Dr. Kennedy compared BBI to other compounds in soy, including genistein and phytic acid. In terms of tumor inhibition, BBI appeared to offer the best result in many different animal studies for many different cancer sites. For example, in rats fed a carcinogen known to induce colon cancer, adding BBI concentrate to their diet suppressed the formation of tumors in

100 percent of the animals. In mice fed a carcinogen known to induce liver cancer, BBI suppressed the formation of tumors by 71 percent. Results such as these have led Dr. Kennedy to believe that BBI is *the* anticancer compound in soy. In fact, she notes that since most of the cancer studies on other compounds in soy have been done using whole food or compounds containing several different phytochemicals, it is possible that BBI alone is responsible for soy's anticancer activity. Obviously, further studies are desperately needed to determine which if any compounds are effective against cancer. Dr. Kennedy is conducting human cancer-prevention trials using BBI in people at high risk of developing cancer. The results of her study may help answer some of the questions surrounding BBI, and other potential anticancer compounds in soy.

We don't know yet which compounds in soy may be anticarcinogenic. Is it BBI? Is it genistein? Is it phytic acid, or is it saponins? Is it some compound that scientists have yet to discover? Or do these compounds work together to thwart the spread of cancer at different stages? It may take decades for scientists to unravel this mystery. In the meantime, you can reap the benefits of these compounds by eating soy foods!

Four

Heart and Soy

Heart disease is the number one killer of men and women in the United States, accounting for 40 percent of all deaths. But in Japan, death from heart disease is rare. Consider the following statistics for 1991, the latest figures available:

- In the United States, 487 men and 232 women per 100,000 died of heart disease.

- In Japan, only 238 men and 121 women per 100,000 succumb to heart disease, roughly half the rate of the United States.

In fact, Japan has the lowest rate in the world for death from heart disease for men, and the second lowest for women. (The mortality rate from heart disease is slightly lower for women in France.) Why is the mortality rate of heart disease so much higher in the United States than in Japan? What are the Japanese doing right, and what are we doing wrong? Once again, the traditional Japanese low-fat, soy-based diet appears to be a major factor. In fact, recent studies show that soy may have some unique properties that make it a potent "heart protector."

1. Researchers have isolated compounds in soy that may directly prevent heart disease by altering blood lipid levels.

2. A soy-based diet may indirectly protect against heart disease because it tends to be lower in fat than food from animal sources. (Studies show that a high-fat diet is a major risk factor for heart disease.)

To fully understand the role of soy in protecting against heart disease, it's important to know exactly what heart disease is and how it develops.

The ABCs of Heart Disease

Atherosclerosis   Atherosclerosis is a progressive disease that often begins in childhood and can lead to coronary artery disease, the cause of most heart attacks. In atherosclerosis, the arteries delivering blood and oxygen to the heart become clogged with plaque, a yellowish, waxy substance. Plaque starts off as fatty streaks in the arteries—in the United States these fatty streaks can appear in children as young as ten years old! Eventually the mass or plaque can become big enough to close off the artery. A reduction in the flow of oxygen and blood to the heart can cause angina, or chest pain. A heart attack occurs when the heart muscle dies or is damaged owing to a lack of nourishment. In some cases, severe atherosclerosis can weaken the artery, resulting in a stretched-out portion called an *aneurysm,* which can cause a rupture in the wall.

There are several theories about what causes atherosclerosis. One theory—called the *injury response theory*—suggests that atherosclerosis begins as a result of an injury to the endothelium, the protective layer around the lumen, the inner core of the artery. In this case, an injury means anything that disturbs the normal function of the cell. For instance, an injury to a cell could be caused by an excess amount of fat or lipids in the blood, which could somehow injure the endothelium. Another theory speculates that plaque is similar to a cancerous tumor that grows wildly out of control. Some people believe that a chemical or virus may trigger this uncontrolled growth. However, there is strong evidence that atherosclerosis is directly related to the balance between particular types of lipids or fat in the blood.

Blood Lipids   Lipids are a form of fat found in the blood. *Fat* has become a dirty word as of late, yet it is essential for life. In fact, a woman's body may be composed of from 25 to 35 percent fatty tissue; a man's body has only about 10 percent less. Fat is an important source of energy. Body fat protects and insulates body organs; it carries fat-soluble vitamins through the body; and it is essential for the production of sex organs. Blood is basically water, and since oil and water don't mix, fat travels through the blood stream on molecules called *lipoproteins.*

Cholesterol   Cholesterol is a lipid that is produced by the liver and is present in foods of animal origin, such as meat and full-fat dairy products. Since cholesterol is basically a fat, it is carried through the body on a lipoprotein. Cholesterol is used by the cells for energy, cell repair, manufacture of sex hormones, and other important jobs.

High-density lipoprotein (HDL) is often called "good cho-lesterol" because it helps rid the body of excess cholesterol. Low-density lipoprotein (LDL), the body's major carrier of cholesterol, is often called "bad cholesterol" because it is be-lieved to be responsible for the formation of plaque. Cells have special binders or receptors that latch on to LDL as they need it. When the cells have enough cholesterol, they stop produc-ing receptors, allowing the LDL to circulate in the bloodstream. Many researchers believe that too much LDL in the blood can cause injury to the artery wall, triggering the formation of plaque.

Diet What does the food we eat have to do with the level of cholesterol in our blood? There is overwhelming evidence that atherosclerosis may be a self inflicted disease.

The Diet Connection

After World War II, when the rate of heart disease continued to soar in Western countries such as the United States, re-searchers began to wonder why certain nationalities appeared to be immune to this problem. Although many scientists be-lieved that a tendency to develop heart disease was genetic (an easy explanation as to why certain nationalities appeared to be immune), others weren't so sure. Researchers began to seriously consider other possible factors. Diet seemed the most striking and consistent difference: In countries where the intake of fat was high—particularly in the form of satu-rated fat from meat or dairy products—deaths from heart disease soared. However, in countries where fat intake was low and the diet was high in vegetables and grain, the rate of heart disease was also low. A major study of nineteen coun-tries by the World Health Organization showed a direct re-lationship among fat intake, blood cholesterol levels, and incidence of heart disease. In this study, researchers found that in countries where people consumed the highest amount of fat in their diets, the average cholesterol level was above 250 mg/dl, nearly one hundred points higher than in countries with low fat intakes. In addition, the countries with the highest cholesterol levels also had the highest rate of heart disease.

Many researchers clung to the belief that some lucky people must be genetically predisposed to low cholesterol levels and low risk of heart disease. However, the on-going Ni-Hon-San Study, which began in 1965, showed that the problem was not in our genes but in what we were putting in our mouths. In this now-famous study, researchers observed the diet of three groups of Japanese men. The first group lived in Japan and ate the traditional Japanese diet consisting of 7 percent saturated fat daily. The second group was men who had moved to Honolulu, where their eating habits became somewhat more Americanized (consuming about 12 percent saturated fat daily). The third group was men who moved to San Francisco, where they began eating the typical American diet, gorging on 14 percent saturated fat daily. Ten years later, the men who had stayed in Japan had the lowest cholesterol levels and the healthiest hearts. Those who went to Honolulu had cholesterol levels that were 12 percent higher than the men living in Japan and had a higher rate of heart disease. But the Japanese in San Francisco fared the poorest: their cholesterol levels were 21 percent higher than the men in Japan and they had the highest rate of heart disease. Since then, numerous studies have confirmed the links among fat intake, cholesterol levels, and heart disease.

There is no doubt that some foods can promote high blood cholesterol and that other foods can lower cholesterol. Many studies have shown that soy is a potent cholesterol buster. In fact, there have been hundreds of studies examining the effect of various forms of soy on blood lipid levels in both animals and people. Most have shown that soy can play a significant role in lowering cholesterol levels.

Soy and Cholesterol

In the 1940s, researchers began studying the effects of plant and animal protein on cholesterol levels and atherosclerosis in animals. In one groundbreaking study, laboratory rabbits were fed a cholesterol-free diet containing 38 percent protein primarily from casein, a milk product. Despite the cholesterol-free regimen, the rabbits on casein eventually developed high cholesterol and severe atherosclerosis of the aorta, the artery delivering blood to the heart. However, when researchers replaced the casein with soy flour, the cholesterol levels remained low and the rabbits remained well.

In a more recent study involving rabbits, researchers compared the effect of feeding the animals either isolated soy protein or a mixture of casein and soy protein. Equal parts of casein and soy protein produced the same results as the soy protein alone, a significant finding because it showed that soy protein was able to counteract the negative effect of casein. In later studies involving other animals, casein was shown to produce higher cholesterol levels than soy protein. The results of these and other animal studies encouraged researchers to test the effects of soy on humans.

One of the world's leading authorities on soy and cholesterol, C. R. Sirtori, of the University of Milan, has performed many studies using soy protein on patients with high cholesterol. For example, one study involved patients with high blood-cholesterol levels who were put on a standard low-fat, low-cholesterol diet for three months. Although the patients showed some reduction in cholesterol, more was needed. The animal protein in their diet was then replaced with soy protein to determine if soy could further cut their cholesterol. The results were dramatic: After three weeks on the textured soy protein, the patients showed an average 21 percent decrease in total cholesterol. However, those kept on the standard low-fat diet who were still eating animal protein did not experience a drop in cholesterol.

In a similar experiment, patients with high cholesterol were given soy protein instead of animal protein along with an additional 500 milligrams of cholesterol daily in the form of egg powder. Interestingly, despite the added cholesterol, the group showed a dramatic decline in total cholesterol levels. In other words, the addition of cholesterol to the diet did not appear to interfere with the ability of soy to cut cholesterol levels.

Soy also appears to reduce cholesterol in patients with normal cholesterol levels, although not as dramatically as in patients with high cholesterol. Under the direction of K. K. Carroll of the University of Western Ontario, researchers examined the effect of soy protein on women with normal blood cholesterol. Female students were put on two different dietary protocols. The first consisted of a normal, well-balanced diet in which protein came from both animals and plants; the second was a normal standard diet with one important exception: the protein portion was derived from soy products. Meat was replaced with soy analogs, and milk was replaced with soy milk. The fat composition of the diet (roughly 40 percent of the total daily calories were derived from fat) remained the same on both regimes. While on soy protein, the students' average cholesterol levels dropped by about 5 percent. The researchers noted that although soy protein appears to work more dramatically in people with elevated cholesterol levels, it also worked reasonably well in people with normal blood lipid levels.

Soy can also reduce cholesterol in children. In rare cases children are born with a genetic tendency to develop extremely high cholesterol. In a recent study involving eleven children with very high cholesterol, researchers found that isolated soy protein could reduce blood cholesterol levels and LDL, or "bad cholesterol," levels more effectively than the standard low-fat diet. For two months the children ate a low-fat, low-cholesterol diet, resulting in a 14 percent drop in total cholesterol and a 17 percent drop in LDL cholesterol. When isolated soy protein replaced the animal protein in their diet, the cholesterol levels dropped even further (32 percent from the start of the diet) and LDL cholesterol fell an additional 20 percent to a 37 percent total reduction. This study is extremely important because if their cholesterol levels went unchecked, these children could be at an extremely high risk of developing heart disease.

Until recently, researchers believed that when it came to lowering cholesterol with soy, it was all or nothing. In other words, in order for soy to work, you had to replace all the animal protein in the diet with vegetable protein. However, a study by Susan Potter, Ph.D., at the University of Illinois at Urbana-Champaign, showed that a little bit of soy can go a long way. Dr. Potter tested four different dietary regimens on twenty-six men with mildly elevated cholesterol levels. All the men were put on a standard low-fat (under 30 percent of daily calories) and low-cholesterol (under 300 milligrams daily) diet. For four consecutive four-week periods, the men substituted half their normal protein intake with baked goods containing 50 grams (roughly 2 ounces) of either soy protein and soy fiber from soy flour; isolated soy protein and soy cotyledon flour; pure isolated soy protein or nonfat dried milk. The researchers found that out of all the dietary protocols, the isolated soy protein worked the best, resulting in a 12 percent drop in total cholesterol and a 11.5 percent drop in LDL, or "bad cholesterol." Based on this study, the researchers concluded that "the fact that a significant reduction was obtained by consuming only 50 g [grams] soy protein/d [daily] sets a practical and achievable goal that would be beneficial in the treatment and prevention of high blood cholesterol and coronary artery disease."

Follow-up studies by Dr. Potter's group showed that even 25 grams of soy protein daily could result in a significant reduction in cholesterol in men with elevated cholesterol levels, though not as much a reduction as those who had 50 grams daily.

How Soy Does It

No one knows the precise mechanism by which soy lowers cholesterol, however here are some interesting theories:

Antioxidant Role   According to the "injury" theory of atherosclerosis, something occurs in the arterial wall that alters the behavior of normal cells. Many researchers believe that the injury may involve the oxidation of LDL cholesterol caused by free radicals, or unstable oxygen molecules. Based on this theory, after LDL cholesterol is oxidized it may attract scavenger cells that gobble up the LDL and form foam cells, thus beginning the formation of plaque. Recent studies show a direct correlation between vitamin E and C intake—both potent antioxidants—and lower cholesterol levels. In fact, one major study involving male medical professionals showed that those who took a vitamin E supplement had a 40 percent reduced risk of having a heart attack.

A handful of studies suggest that soy may also have antioxidant properties. A team of Japanese researchers from Hirosaki University School of Medicine recently tested this theory on laboratory rabbits. In their study, they checked the effect of soy milk on LDL cholesterol in laboratory rats. First, they fed the rabbits a standard Oriental diet with added cholesterol; in the second phase of the study, they divided the rabbits into groups: one group received the same diet but were also given Probucol, a known antioxidant. The other group received the same diet, however they were given additional soy milk. The result: the rate of lipid peroxidation fell dramatically on both diets, and so did cholesterol levels. In fact, the soy worked even better than the Probucol in preventing LDL oxidation! The researchers, who reported their results in the *Annals of the New York Academy of Sciences,* concluded, "Thus, because soy proteins decreased the production of oxidized and deformed LDL, they are very useful in preventing the development of atherosclerotic diseases [hardening of the arteries]."

Genistein Role   Genistein, an isoflavone found in soy, is believed to inhibit the action of enzymes that may promote cell growth and migration. Some researchers speculate that by blocking the action of these enzymes, genistein may also prevent the growth of cells that form plaque deposits in arteries, much the same way that genistein may prevent the growth of tumors.

Hormone Effect   Researchers suggested that the particular combination of amino acids found in soy may alter an important step in the manufacture of cholesterol. Some studies have shown that after eating soy protein, blood glucagon levels rise (glucagon is a hormone released by the pancreas). Researchers speculate that a shift in glucagon levels may somehow alter the activity of HMG Co A reductase (Coenzyme A), which is necessary for the synthesis of cholesterol. Interestingly, the cholesterol-lowering drug Mevacor also works by interfering with Coenzyme A activity.

Estrogenic Effect   Some researchers speculate that the phytoestrogens in soy may exert an estrogenic effect on the body that somehow lowers cholesterol. Estrogen plays a major role in the way lipids are produced, handled, broken down, and eliminated from the body. Studies show that after menopause, when estrogen levels drop in women, cholesterol levels typically rise along with a woman's risk of developing coronary artery disease (CAD). However, women who take estrogen-replacement therapy experience a dramatic drop in LDL and a rise in HDL. Other studies have shown that estrogen increases the number of LDL receptors in cells, which means that less cholesterol is left circulating in the blood. All of these factors lead some researchers to wonder whether soy's ability to lower LDLs and cholesterol is related to its estrogen activity.

Thyroid Connection   Animal studies have found that soy can raise blood plasma levels of thyroxine, a hormone produced by the thyroid gland, while at the same time lowering blood cholesterol. In fact, studies have shown that an increase in thyroxine always precedes the drop in cholesterol. People who have underactive thyroid glands (hypothyroidism) tend to have high levels of blood cholesterol. Therefore, researchers hypothesize that soy may somehow stimulate the thyroid gland to produce more hormone, which in turn lowers blood cholesterol.

Binding Factor Some researchers suggest that soy somehow binds with bile in the intestine and is excreted in the feces. The liver compensates by producing more bile salts, which requires cholesterol, thus reducing the amount of circulating cholesterol.

Amino Acid Composition Soy protein has lower levels of certain essential amino acids, such as lysine and methionine, than animal protein. Studies have shown that when lysine is added to a soy diet, the level of LDL rises. Researchers speculate that the particular mix of amino acids in soy may somehow prevent the formation of plaque.

Phytic Acid Effect A chelating agent that binds to iron, phytic acid increases copper absorption in the body. In several studies, copper deficiency has been associated with high cholesterol.

Lowering Your Cholesterol with Soy

According to the American Heart Association, nearly 95 million American adults have blood cholesterol levels over 200 mg/dl and 37 million have levels over 240 mg/dl. According to the National Cholesterol Education Program, cholesterol levels should be 200 mg/dl or less. If your cholesterol level is high, you should talk to your doctor or nutritionist about whether you should try to reduce it.

If you do need to cut your cholesterol, soy and other natural aids can help. However, there is no magic bullet that can cut cholesterol regardless of what you eat; diet is also very important. Anyone who needs to cut cholesterol should adopt the so-called prudent, or heart-healthy, diet.

1. Depending on your weight and activity level, you may have to cut back on calories. Talk to your physician or natural healer about determining your ideal weight.

2. Reduce your daily fat intake to no more than 20 percent of total calories (in some cases, you may have to go even lower).

3. Consume no more than 10 percent of your calories in the form of saturated fat. Saturated fat stimulates the body to produce cholesterol.

4. Watch your meat portions. Meat is a major source of saturated fat. Portions should be no bigger than 3 or 4 ounces after cooking, about the size of a deck of cards. Stick to lean cuts of meat, chicken or fish daily.

5. Limit your cholesterol intake to 300 milligrams daily.

Although this list may sound restrictive, there are hundreds of foods that are high in taste but low in fat and cholesterol. Consult a nutritional counselor to help you devise a diet that agrees with your palate as well as your heart.

In addition to the prudent diet, add soy protein as an excellent cholesterol buster. Based on the University of Illinois study, about 50 grams of isolated soy protein daily (roughly the amount in one cup) can cut cholesterol levels by 12 percent. (The soy protein must replace about half your normal daily protein intake. In order to make sure you're cutting down on protein, eat your soy product first. In addition, if you're adding 50 grams soy protein to your diet, restrict your intake of meat to one 3- or 4-ounce serving daily, cooked weight.)

There are several ways to get your daily quotient of soy protein.

1. Sprinkle 1 to 3 tablespoons of isolated soy protein on your food. Flavorless ISP can be used on cereal, yogurt, or fruit salad, or in soups and sauces..

2. You can drink it. St. Louis–based Nutritious Foods, Inc., is marketing beverage powders and food ingredients called Take Care that contain 20 grams of soy protein in the form of SUPRO brand isolated soy protein, a product developed by Protein Technologies International. SUPRO has been used in many studies on cholesterol reduction. As of this writing, it contains the highest level of soy protein of any product on the market. The instant beverage powder also contains 20 milligrams of genistein and comes flavored or plain. (For information on where to buy it, see page 237.) You can also concoct your own beverage using soy protein isolate, which can be purchased in most natural food stores. Soy protein isolate contains 13 grams of soy protein per 2 tablespoons. Soy protein isolate can be mixed with juice or fruit and blended into a protein-packed drink or soup for breakfast or lunch.

The following recipes using Take Care were created by Susan W. Reeves, R.D., L.D., of Little Rock, Arkansas, for Nutritious Foods.

Tutti-fruitti

1 serving (20 g soy protein)

1 cup skim milk

½ banana

½ cup fresh or frozen unsweetened strawberries (if frozen, do not thaw)

2 scoops strawberry flavored Take Care Nutritious Beverage Powder, High-Protein Formula

1 bottle (10 ounces) cherry-flavored sparkling water, chilled

Combine first 4 ingredients in container of an electric blender, cover and process until smooth. Pour the fruit mixture into a 16-ounce glass and stir in water.

PER SERVING Calories: 275   Fat: 2 g
             Saturated fat: 0   Fiber: 1 g
             Cholesterol: 4 mg   Calcium: 1017 mg
             Iron: 4.4 mg

Pineapple Mock Daiquiri

1 serving (20 g soy protein)

1 can (6 ounces) pineapple juice, chilled

2 tablespoons lime juice, chilled

2 scoops plain Take Care Nutritious Beverage Powder, High-Protein Formula

¼ teaspoon rum extract

5 ice cubes

Combine all ingredients in container of an electric blender. Cover and process until smooth. Pour into a 12-ounce glass.

PER SERVING Calories: 201   Fat: 1g
             Saturated fat: less than 1 g   Fiber: less than 1 g
             Cholesterol: 0   Calcium: 335 mg
             Iron: 2 mg

Raspberry Cream

1 serving (20 g soy protein)

1 cup of frozen unsweetened raspberries, thawed

1 cup fat-free vanilla ice cream

½ cup skim milk

*2 scoops plain Take Care Nutritious Beverage Powder, High-
    Protein Formula*

In a blender or a food processor fitted with a steel blade, process raspberries until pureed. Strain raspberries; reserve puree and discard seeds. Return raspberry puree to the blender, add remaining ingredients and process until smooth. Spoon into a 16-ounce glass.

PER SERVING Calories: 364   Fat: 2 g
             Saturated fat: Less than 1 g   Fiber: 4 g
             Cholesterol: 10 mg   Calcium: 878 mg
             Iron: 4 mg

Caramel Hot Cocoa

1 serving (20 g soy protein)

1 envelop sugar-free hot cocoa mix

*2 scoops chocolate Take Care Nutritious Beverage Powder,
    High-Protein Formula*

⅔ cup very hot water

1 tablespoon caramel ice cream topping

Place cocoa mix and Take Care in a large mug. Add hot water,
whisk until smooth. Stir in ice cream topping.

PER SERVING Calories: 250   Fat: 1.5 g

Saturated fat: 0   Fiber: 0

Cholesterol: 5 mg   Calcium: 300 mg

Iron: 1.4 mg

Potato Soup

4 servings (15 g soy protein each)

2½ cups peeled, cubed baking potatoes

2 cups water

⅓ cup sliced carrot

¼ cup sliced celery

¼ cup chopped onion

6 scoops plain Take Care Nutritious Food Ingredient

1½ cups evaporated skim milk

2 tablespoons chopped green onion

1 tablespoon chopped fresh parsley

1 teaspoon salt

½ teaspoon ground white pepper

Dash of hot pepper sauce

1. Combine first 5 ingredients in a medium saucepan and bring to boil. Reduce heat and simmer uncovered for 20 minutes or until vegetables are tender. Drain well, reserving 1½ cups of cooking liquid.

2. In a food processor fitted with a steel blade, process half of the vegetable mixture, half of the reserved cooking liquid, and the Take Care until smooth. Pour mixture into saucepan. Repeat with remaining vegetable mixture and cooking liquid. Add remaining ingredients to pureed vegetables mixture in pan. Cook over medium heat for 5 minutes or until heated through, stirring occasionally. Serve hot.

PER SERVING Calories: 194   Fat: 1 g
             Saturated Fat: Less than 1 g   Fiber: Less than 1 g
             Cholesterol: 4 mg   Calcium: 819 mg
             Iron: 3 mg

Red Pepper Bisque

2 servings (10 g soy protein each)

½ cup skim milk

1 jar (7 ounces) roasted sweet red peppers, undrained

2 scoops plain Take Care Nutritious Food Ingredient

2 tablespoons Neufchatel cheese, softened

2 teaspoons white wine vinegar

1 teaspoon salt

½ teaspoon prepared horseradish

⅛ teaspoon ground red pepper

Chopped parsley to garnish

Place all ingredients except parsley in a blender or food processor fitted with a steel blade and process until smooth. Transfer to small saucepan. Stirring occasionally, cook over medium heat until heated through. Spoon into individual serving bowls and garnish with chopped parsley if desired.

PER SERVING Calories: 145   Fat: 6 g
             Saturated fat: 0 g   Fiber: 1 g
             Cholesterol: 11 g   Calcium: 436 mg
             Iron: 2 mg

Part II

SOY FOR SPECIAL NEEDS

Five

Just for Women: Rx for Menopause and Osteoporosis

When you talk about menopause in the United States, the first thing that comes to mind are hot flashes, the quintessential symptom of the "change of life." Interestingly, there is no word in Japanese to describe a hot flash. In fact, many studies show that most Japanese women never experience a hot flash, and, in fact, complain of far fewer unpleasant symptoms of menopause than do Western women.

A recent study by Canadian researchers of Japanese women and menopause reported that "the hot flush or flash, seen in the West as the sine qua non of the menopausal woman, were mentioned by only 12 of the 105 women and no one talked about night sweats." In another study, researchers compared the menopausal experiences of Japanese, Canadian, and U.S. women. The Japanese women had far fewer physical complaints than did the Western women. Nearly 35 percent of U.S. women and 31 percent of Canadian women reported having hot flashes, versus only 12.4 percent of the Japanese women. More than 38.1 percent of the American women complained of a lack of energy; only 6 percent of the Japanese women had the same complaint. More than 35 percent of the U.S. women complained of depression, only 10.3 of the Japanese women said they felt depressed. In fact, researchers reported that few Japanese women were on any medication (hormone replacement therapy) for menopause. However, Japanese women did use more herbs and herbal teas.

The studies comparing menopause in Japan to menopause in the West generated much controversy. Some sociologists contended that Japanese women couldn't feel so much better than Western women; rather, they were exhibiting Asian stoicism—in other words, they felt rotten but weren't complaining about it! However, *Lancet*, a leading British medical journal, published a letter by Dr. Herman Adlercreutz, a major researcher in the field of phytoestrogens, in which he suggested that Japanese women may actually have fewer menopausal symptoms because of their diets. Dr. Adlercreutz pointed out that Japanese women eat high amounts of soy foods, and soy foods contain isoflavones. "All isoflavonoids are weak oestrogens [sic] and such high amounts could have biological effects, especially in postmenopausal women with low oestrogen levels. High levels of isoflavonoid phyto-oestrogens may partly explain why hot flushes and other menopausal symptoms are so infrequent in Japanese women."

Although the precise cause of hot flashes is not known, they are probably caused by hormonal fluctuations at menopause, when estrogen levels dip and the body compensates for the loss by producing more luteninizing hormone (LH) to stimulate the ovaries. It's possible that if the phytoestrogens in soy bind to estrogen receptors that would otherwise remain empty, the body may be fooled into thinking it has enough estrogen.

Soy may also help relieve another discomfort associated with menopause: thinning of the vaginal walls. After estrogen levels drop, the lining of the vagina begins to thin, which can result in painful intercourse and a potential for developing infections. Soy may prevent this from happening. A recent study described in the *British Medical Journal* attempted to see whether eating foods rich in phytoestrogens could prevent thinning of the vaginal wall. Postmenopausal women were given three different foods—soy flour, linseed oil, and red clover sprouts—daily for two weeks each. During the soy period, there was a greater increase in the number of cells in the vaginal epithelium than during the other food periods. The researchers concluded that "patterns of food intake may modulate the severity of the menopause as it is an oestrogen deficiency state" (*BMJ*, 301, October 20, 1990).

Soy for Strong Bones

Preliminary research suggests that soy foods may be a useful tool in maintaining strong bones. This is good news, especially for people at risk of developing osteoporosis, a disease characterized by a thinning or wearing down of bone tissue, which leaves the bones vulnerable to fractures and breaks. Osteoporosis is a virtual epidemic among the elderly, especially older women. In fact, about 15 million Americans—75 percent of them women—have osteoporosis. As the population ages, that number is expected to soar.

Osteoporosis is a disease of aging. In young people, bone is constantly being produced by the body. The creation of new bone is a complex process involving the interaction of minerals such as calcium and potassium, and hormones such as estrogen in women and testosterone in men, and vitamin D. However, at around age forty or so, women especially begin to use up more bone than they can produce. So do men; however, men have more bone mass to begin with, and typically do not lose as much as do women. In fact, on average, postmenopausal women lose about 5 percent of their bone mass annually, the process being accelerated by a drop in their estrogen levels.

Not all women are at equal risk of developing osteoporosis. Caucasian and Asian women—especially those who are thin boned and petite—run a much greater risk of osteoporosis than women of African descent.

Although few people consider osteoporosis to be as serious as a disease as heart disease or cancer, in reality it is a leading killer of women. Typically, an older woman falls and injures her hip, a common site for injury. About 15 percent of all women with hip injuries die shortly after being injured. Within a year, nearly a third will die owing to complications such as a blood clot. Hip injuries are also a major reason why older women wind up in nursing homes.

Paradoxically, even though Asian women are small boned, they have far fewer hip injuries than do Caucasian women. In fact, Japanese women have roughly half the hip injuries of U.S. women, and women in Hong Kong and Singapore fare even better. What's even more mysterious is the fact that Asian women consume far less dietary calcium than do U.S. women.

Exercise may be one of the reasons why Asian women are spared hip injuries. For example, in traditional Japanese homes people sit on the floor. Having to get up and down dozens of times a day may help a woman develop strong muscles and bones in the hip region. However, diet may also play a small role in helping to reduce the rate of hip fractures.

Even though Asian women eat less bone-building calcium, their bodies may better utilize the calcium that they do eat. For one thing, Asian women eat less protein than Western women. Several studies have shown that protein in general, and animal protein in particular, increases urinary excretion of calcium, which means that the body has less calcium to draw upon if it needs it. Although the amount of calcium excreted is very small, over a lifetime it could have a significant effect on available calcium, and that could make a difference in terms of bone mass.

In addition, studies have shown that consumption of soy protein results in far less urinary calcium excretion than does animal protein. In one study conducted at the University of Texas, researchers found that people who ate soy protein lost 50 percent less calcium through their urine than if they ate animal protein. Since most Asian women eat more soy products than U.S. women, they could be retaining more calcium even though they consume less.

Other studies suggest that the isoflavones in soy may help retain bone mass. Two recent studies headed by John Anderson at the University of North Carolina investigated the effect of genistein on bone mass in rats who had their ovaries removed to eliminate their natural supply of estrogen, and on young animals who were still growing. In one study, the rats were lactating, which increased their calcium demand; the other study involved young rats who were not fully grown and, therefore, still needed to build bone. In both studies, rats were fed a daily supplement of genistein at varying strengths. Another group of similar rats were fed a daily supplement of Premarin, a synthetic estrogen given to postmenopausal women to prevent osteoporosis. The results show that the low-dose genistein was able to prevent bone loss almost as well as the Premarin. Notes Dr. Anderson, "It looks promising that genistein may have some preventive effect on bone loss," but he cautions that more studies need to be done.

Dr. Anderson speculates that genistein's possible effects on bone may be due to its weak estrogenic properties. Like other cells in the body, bone cells have estrogen receptors, but far fewer than reproductive cells. As women become menopausal and their estrogen levels drop, these receptors lay fallow. It's probable that the plant estrogens in soy may bind to these receptors, which might help to maintain bone tissue much the same way as do real estrogens. However, since plant estrogens are weaker, they probably are not as effective. Dr. Anderson also points out that although Japanese women may have lower rates of hip fractures, osteoporosis of the spine is a common problem, probably owing to their naturally thin bones. Nevertheless, Dr. Anderson believes, "Our studies suggest that Japanese women may have a lifetime of protection of retaining a bit more bone at all sites because of this dietary soy factor."

Soy may indeed prove to be a "bone-sparing" food. Given the results of these early studies, it makes sense to include soy food as part of an anti-osteoporosis diet; however, it should be used along with other bone builders, including the following:

1. Calcium. Calcium is critical for strong bones. Low-fat yogurt, tofu made with calcium sulfate, canned salmon with bones, almonds, fortified cereals, and leafy green vegetables are excellent sources of this mineral.

2. Vitamin D. Without the sunshine vitamin, calcium cannot be absorbed by the body. To bone up on vitamin D, eat fortified dairy products and fatty fish.

3. Estrogen-replacement therapy (ERT). In women who are at high risk of developing osteoporosis, hormone-replacement therapy after menopause may be the only way to save their bones. However, synthetic hormones should not be taken lightly; studies show that there is an increase in breast cancer and endometrial cancers among women who are on ERT. Women with a family history of cancer, stroke, or high blood pressure should carefully evaluate ERT with their physicians before taking synthetic hormones.

4. Exercise. Regular weight-bearing exercise is one of the proven ways to maintain bone mass. Walking at least two miles a day, practicing yoga, or pumping iron at the gym are all bone builders.

5. Boron. This mineral, found in grapes and dried fruit, helps raise levels of blood estrogens in postmenopausal women, which may help retain calcium.

Avoid these bone breakers:

1. Caffeine increases calcium excretion. Watch the coffee and the caffeinated colas!

2. Smoking increases your risk of developing osteoporosis.

3. Excess alcohol interferes with mineral absorption.

4 Phosphates, found in many soft drinks, can deplete calcium levels.

Six

Just for Men: Rx for Prostate Problems

The prostate is a small, walnut-size gland located between the bladder and the penis, above the rectum; it surrounds the beginning of the urethra (the tube that carries urine from the bladder to outside of the body). The prostate gland produces semen, the fluid that carries sperm. At some time in his life, nearly every man experiences some problem with his prostate. In many cases, these problems may be preventable through proper diet and nutrition. Soy food in particular is good for maintaining a healthy prostate, and there are other herbs and supplements that may also be useful.

Prostatitis

About one in five men will get an inflammation of their prostate, called prostatitis. The symptoms include pain or difficulty during urination, blood or pus in the urine, fever, chills, or pain in the lower back. (If you experience any of these symptoms, see your doctor.) Prostatitis can be caused by any number of factors including an infection, too much (or too little) sexual activity, dehydration, irritation to the area owing to bicycle or horseback riding, or prolonged sitting. Coffee and alcohol may also be irritating to the prostate. Prostatitis may be treated with antibiotics (if the cause is an infection), bed rest, and warm baths.

Prostatitis may also be aggravated by estrogen, which promotes cell growth. Soy food, which can dampen the effects of estrogen, may help prevent the proliferation of inflammatory cells that can lead to prostatitis. In one study, three groups of adult male rats, all prone to developing prostatitis, were fed different diets. One group was fed a diet in which soy was the protein source; the second was fed a soy-free diet. The third group was fed laboratory rat chow that included soy protein. After eleven weeks there was a marked increase in prostatitis among the rats fed a soy-free diet, and a dramatic decline in the amount of phytoestrogens excreted in their urine. The researchers concluded, "This study suggests that soy of dietary source may play a protective role against the pathogenesis of the prostate."

Men of all ages should take extra zinc. There are heavy concentrations of zinc in the male prostate gland. In fact, mild prostate deficiency can lead to a low sperm count. All men should eat foods that are rich in zinc, including oysters, brewer's yeast, wheat germ, and pumpkin seeds. (Lamb chops and liver are also high in zinc, but they are also high in fat. If you eat them, do so sparingly.) Men should also take a daily zinc supplement of up to 60 milligrams of zinc gluconate.

Drinking plenty of fluids can also help to keep your prostate healthy.

Benign Prostate Hypertrophy

Nearly half of all men over fifty develop benign prostate hypertrophy (BPH) or an enlarged prostate. (In severe cases, the prostate can grow to the size of an orange.) Symptoms include an increase in the urge to urinate, especially at night; incomplete emptying of the bladder, which can lead to infection; or pain with erection or orgasm. A new medication has been used to treat this problem successfully in many men, although surgery may be required in severe cases.

Enlargement of the prostate may be caused by an accumulation of testosterone. Since estrogen may trigger the production of male hormones, by moderating estrogen activity soy food may help prevent prostatic enlargement.

Natural healers use the berries from the saw palmetto tree to treat an enlarged prostate. In fact, in Germany, saw palmetto is recognized as an effective over-the-counter drug for this problem. Saw palmetto capsules are sold in natural food stores and herb shops. Take one capsule up to three times daily.

Prostate Cancer

Up until recently, prostate cancer was a taboo subject; few men wanted to even think about it, much less talk about it. However, the deaths of several prominent men from prostate cancer, including Frank Zappa, Steve Ross, Telly Savalas, and Bill Bixby, have increased public awareness about this potentially lethal disease.

Next to skin cancer, prostate cancer is the second most common form of cancer to strike men. In 1993, about 165,000 new cases of prostate cancer were diagnosed, and 35,000 men died from this disease. Most new cases of prostate cancer occur in men over fifty-five. African-American men are particularly prone to prostate cancer. (One out of nine African-American men will get prostate cancer vs. one out of eleven white men.)

Because of the prevalence of prostate cancer, the American Cancer Society recommends that by age forty, every man have an annual physical examination that includes an internal exam of the prostate and rectum. (The physician can feel the prostate by inserting a gloved finger in the rectum.) Through this physical examination the physician can detect whether the prostate is enlarged, infected, or shows tumor growth. The American Cancer Society also recommends that men over fifty have a prostate-specific antigen blood test to detect any early cancers. If the physical exam or blood test is abnormal, follow-up tests including ultrasound are required before a diagnosis can be made. Needless to say, if you have any pain during urination, or blood or pus in the urine, or any other sign that something isn't right, you should see your doctor.

Prostate cancer can't be cured but it can be controlled. Standard cancer treatments, including surgery and chemotherapy, are used to prevent the cancer from spreading to other organs. In fact, if it's caught early the prognosis is quite good. Recent studies have shown that in older men with slow-growing tumors, treatment may not be required. In fact, many members of the medical community now advocate a "watchful waiting" period in which the cancer is monitored. If the progress is slow, in some cases the risk of treatment could be greater than leaving the cancer alone.

Diet may play a role in prostate cancer. Japanese men have the lowest mortality rate from prostate cancer in the world, although their rate of developing prostate cancer is just as high as in the West. Prostate tumors are often hormone sensitive, which means that hormones such as estrogen and testosterone may promote their growth. Soy, a staple of the Japanese diet, may help moderate hormone levels in the body, thus reducing the amount of potent circulating hormones. In addition, in test-tube studies, genistein—an isoflavone in soy—has been shown to inhibit the growth of prostate tumor cells.

Fat may also promote the growth of prostate tumors. A recent study, performed by researchers at Harvard Medical School, of 48,000 men showed that those who ate the most animal fat (red meat, butter, and chicken with skin) had the greatest risk of developing a more advanced form of prostate cancer. In other words, diet didn't seem to help prevent the cancer, but a high-fat diet appears to make it progress more quickly.

In addition, vitamin D may help prevent prostate cancer. Another study showed that men who live in areas with the least amount of ultraviolet (UV) rays have higher rates of prostate cancer than those in areas with higher levels of UV waves. Researchers suspect that vitamin D, a hormone produced in the body after exposure to UV waves, may be a factor in prostate cancer. This is not a carte blanche to go sunbathing— excess exposure to UV waves can cause skin cancer. However, it might be a good idea to increase your consumption of vitamin D–rich foods, including fortified, nonfat dairy products and fatty fish (salmon, mackerel, tuna, anchovies).

Japanese men eat between 40 and 70 milligrams of genistein per day. U.S. men eat less than 1 milligram!

Seven

Kids, Cancer, and Heart Disease

"Teach your children well," was the line of a popular song of the 1970s. But when it comes to health, American adults are not heeding this advice. Recently, the Centers for Disease Control and Prevention surveyed the dietary habits and lifestyle of more than 91,000 American adults to assess their risk of developing heart disease. The results of the study were dismal: only 18 percent of all adults over eighteen were free of the major known risk factors for heart disease (high cholesterol, obesity, high blood pressure, diabetes, physical inactivity, and smoking). In fact, even among the youngest adults—the healthiest group in the survey—fewer than 25 percent were totally risk free. The survey concluded that this study "underscores the need for primary prevention efforts that focus on achieving behavioral changes that prevent the occurrence of risk factors."

Unfortunately, the same risk factors that increase the odds of getting heart disease also increase the odds of developing different forms of cancer. Experts estimate that nearly three-quarters of all cases of coronary artery disease and about half of all cancer cases are directly related to poor diet and nutrition, which can cause problems such as obesity and diabetes. Neither heart disease nor cancer happens overnight. The seeds for these diseases are sown early in life, often during childhood. Study after study verifies that America's children are not eating wisely or well. For example:

- The average child eats a diet in which 35 percent of total daily calories are in the form of fat. The American Heart Association and the American Cancer Society recommend that no more than 30 percent of daily calories come in the form of fat.

- The average child consumes 15 percent of his or her daily calories in the form of saturated fat, yet experts recommend under 10 percent. High levels of dietary saturated fat are associated with both heart disease and cancer.

- America's children are getting fatter. Roughly one in three children are overweight, which increases their odds of developing adult obesity, high blood pressure, and diabetes.

- About 1 percent of all children have a genetic problem that predisposes them to high cholesterol. Yet more than 25 percent of all children have cholesterol levels over 170 mg/dl, which increases their risk of developing heart disease as adults. About 5 percent have cholesterol levels over 200 mg/dl.

- The average child is "fiber starved," eating only half of the recommended amount of grams of fiber daily. Although adults are supposed to have between 20 to 40 grams of fiber daily, children require less depending on their age. To determine the amount of fiber a child requires daily, take his age and add 5 to 10. For example, using this formula, an eight year old should have between 13 and 18 grams of fiber daily.

• Few American children follow the advice of the National Cancer Institute and eat their five daily portions of fruits and vegetables. They are not only cheating themselves out of important vitamins and minerals but are missing out on important phytochemicals that may offer special protection against cancer and heart disease.

• Few American children eat a significant amount of soy food. Asian children excrete high levels of isoflavones such as genistein in their urine; American children excrete virtually none. Isoflavones may offer special protection against cancer and heart disease.

The American Heart Association estimates that 80 million Americans under the age of twenty-one will eventually die of coronary artery disease or stroke. If current trends continue, at least half of them will contract some form of cancer in their lifetime.

The nutritional status of children can have a profound effect on their health as adults. The overweight child is more likely to grow into the overweight adult. And although it may be decades before it turns into heart disease, the first stage of atherosclerosis may start in the late teens, when fatty streaks that may later become raised lesions begin to appear in the coronary arteries of America's young people. (Asian teenagers, who typically are on low-fat diets, may also develop fatty streaks, but they rarely progress to raised lesions and may even disappear.)

Children cannot be blamed for their poor health habits, but their parents can. Children learn by example, and as shown by the survey conducted by the Centers for Disease Control, many parents are not showing their children how to eat right. Christine Williams, M.D., is a pediatrician at the American Health Foundation. She works with children with high cholesterol to help them reduce their cholesterol through dietary intervention. In fact, later this year Dr. Williams will be performing a study to determine if feeding 20 grams of soy protein daily to children in the form of a delicious tofu shake can help reduce cholesterol. (Several studies have shown that soy protein can help reduce blood cholesterol levels in adults and children.) Although cholesterol isn't a problem for most children, Dr. Williams feels that American parents must help their children make constructive changes in their diet, including:

1. Lower saturated fat. Saturated fat is found primarily in foods of animal origin such as meat, eggs, and whole-fat dairy products. Dr. Williams advises parents to reduce the amount of fatty meat in their children's diet. She recommends using soy products as a low-fat source of protein.

2. Lower total fat. Look for opportunities to substitute low-fat products for high-fat ones. Children over two will do fine on reduced-fat milk and dairy products. Throw out the high-fat, high-calorie premium ice cream and buy ice milk or low-fat frozen yogurt instead. Buy low-fat or nonfat salad dressings and baked goods. If your kids like to munch on junk food, try the nonfat chips and reduced-fat and -calorie cookies. Don't forget that fresh fruit is always a good, fat-free option!

3. Increase complex carbohydrates and fiber. When you decrease fat in the diet you also decrease calories because fat is twice as rich in calories as carbohydrates or protein. To compensate for lost fat calories, you should increase dietary intake of complex carbohydrates. This means more pasta, rice, potatoes, crackers, bread, and

cereal. If you choose whole grain products, you will also provide more of the dietary fiber that your child needs.

4. Be persistent. Dr. Williams says that parents often make the mistake of giving up too easily when they try to introduce a new food. According to Dr. Williams, it can take up to six different attempts to introduce a food before a child may like it. So if your child says "yuck," every time you mention a vegetarian pizza or a tofu shake, encourage him or her to taste it, and keep on serving it to other members of your family. It may take a while, but in many cases your child will come around.

5. Be innovative. Try to sneak fruits and vegetables into foods where your children least expect them. Dr. William says that a child who may turn his or her nose up at a serving of carrots may not mind them cooked in a stew or diced in tomato sauce. Fruit and vegetable breads (banana bread, zucchini bread) are also a good way to increase vegetable or fruit consumption without being obvious about it. A tofu or soy milkshake made with fresh fruit is also an excellent way to get kids to eat both soy and fruit!

Eight

Tips for Vegetarians

It used to be that dinner was synonymous with a heaping portion of meat accompanied by a few paltry side dishes. But times have changed. Americans are cutting back on their consumption of animal products. In fact, a record 5 percent of the population—some 12 million people—are total vegetarians. That is, they don't eat any meat, fish, or poultry. Out of this group, some vegetarians abstain from dairy (lactovegetarians) and/or eggs (ovolactovegetarians). What's not counted in this statistic are the millions of other people who have adapted a "quasi-vegetarian lifestyle,"—that is, they eat small amounts of fish or chicken (but may treat themselves to a steak from time to time), using animal protein as a condiment rather than as the focal point of their meals. In fact, many people eat meatless meals several times a week, replacing animal protein with soy, pasta, or legumes and vegetables.

Some people are attracted to total vegetarianism out of purely altruistic reasons: they believe that it is wrong to eat animals. However, many others have become interested in vegetarianism (or quasi-vegetarianism) for health reasons. Study after study confirms that vegetarians are healthier than meat eaters. For instance:

- **Vegetarians measure up**—Vegetarians have lower rates of heart disease, lower blood pressure, and lower rates of many different forms of cancer including colon cancer and breast cancer. For example, one British study found that vegetarians had significantly lower levels of cholesterol than meat eaters, which could result in a 57 percent reduced risk of having a heart attack.

- **Vegetables are good medicine**—Dr. Dean Ornish (author of *Dr. Dean Ornish's Program for Reversing Heart Disease*) found that a vegetarian diet can actually reverse heart disease, often eliminating the need for surgery.

- **The phytochemical factor**—New information about phytochemicals (special compounds in food that may protect against disease) confirms the importance of eating a diet containing a wide variety of plant food, especially soy.

- **High in what you need, low in what you don't** —Sources of plant protein are typically low in fat, especially saturated fat, and high in fiber—just the opposite of animal protein. Few Americans get enough fiber, the indigestible part of the plant that may offer protection against cancer and heart disease. Many Americans get too much saturated fat, which promotes the formation of cholesterol in the body. For example, a lean 3-ounce cooked hamburger contains 23 grams of protein and 7 grams of saturated fat. A 4½-ounce serving of tofu contains 20 grams protein and, depending on whether you use full-fat or nonfat tofu, the amount of saturated fat could range from 2 to 0 grams.

Clearly there are many advantages to going vegetarian, however there are a some problems that may arise with a vegetarian diet.

The Iron Question

Soy contains compounds that can inhibit the absorption of iron, and this may be a problem for some segments of the population. In developing nations, iron deficiency is widespread, although is far less common in the United States. (The RDA for iron is 15 milligrams for women fifteen to fifty; 10 milligrams for women over fifty and men; 15 to 18 milligrams for children.) Some groups, however, may be prone to iron deficiency, including women with heavy menstrual cycles, pregnant women, nursing mothers, adolescents, and children between the ages of six months and four years. If iron levels dip too low, iron deficient anemia could result, a condition characterized by a deficiency in the number of red blood cells and/or a reduction in the number of hemoglobin molecules. Symptoms include fatigue, inability to concentrate, and a susceptibility to infection. Although there's no evidence that vegetarians are more prone to anemia than meat eaters (there are many excellent vegetable sources of iron, especially soybeans and other legumes), meat is still considered the best form of heme iron   that is, the kind of iron that is most easily utilized by the body. For years, nutritionists have worried that people who don't eat meat may not be getting enough iron.

Recent studies should put some of those worries to rest. For example, in one study researchers fed young male students soy protein as their only source of protein for eighty-two days. At the end of the study they found a slight dip in blood iron levels, but not a significant one. In another study soy protein was added to extend ground beef. Researchers found that the addition of soy did not affect iron utilization in any of the children, women, or men included in the study. However, in both studies researchers noted that soy protein should be used in conjunction with ascorbic acid (vitamin C), which helps the body absorb iron better.

On the other hand, too much iron may be more of a problem than too little. In fact, high levels of blood iron have been associated with increased risk of heart disease and cancer.

Watch the B$_{12}$

Vitamin B$_{12}$ is found primarily in animal products, and its deficiency can result in pernicious anemia. In addition, folic acid—another important B vitamin—cannot be utilized without B$_{12}$. Strict vegetarians who avoid dairy and eggs may be prone to B$_{12}$ deficiency. There are some good plant sources of B$_{12}$ including tempeh, fortified cereal, and brewer's yeast. If you don't eat foods containing B$_{12}$, you should take a daily supplement.

The Right Combination

Unlike most other vegetable sources of protein, soy contains all eight essential amino acids that the body cannot produce itself and is high in lysine, an amino acid that is rare in vegetables. Therefore, it is considered a bona fide meat substitute. However, like other vegetable proteins, soy protein is better utilized if accompanied by a complementing protein— that is, a protein source that contains a different combination of amino acids. For example, legumes and grains go well together because they fill in the "amino acid gaps," in each food. Here are some examples of food soy combinations that make complete proteins:

- Tofu lasagna (tofu replaces the ricotta cheese and meat)
- Tofu vegetable stir-fry over brown rice
- Barbecued tempeh with quinoa (a grain that also contains eight essential amino acids)
- Macaroni and "cheese" (made with tofu as a cheese substitute)
- Tofu quiche with a whole wheat pastry crust
- Chili with tofu over rice
- Veggie burgers (made from soy protein) on a whole-grain bun with rice

Caution: Parents who are feeding their children vegetarian diets—especially those who do not use dairy or eggs—must be very careful to ensure that their children are getting enough protein, iron, calcium, and other vitamins and minerals. Many pediatricians believe that a total vegan diet is not appropriate for children. Talk with a nutritionist or family physician about devising a healthful diet for your children.

Part III

NOT BY
SOY ALONE

Nine

Thirty-Seven Miracle Foods from the Pacific Rim

In addition to soy, Asian cuisines are filled with delicious, healthful, low-fat, high-fiber foods, many of which contain important phytochemicals. Here are some foods that you should know about.

Adzuki (Azuki) Beans Next to soybeans, these small red beans are the most common legume in Japanese cooking. Adzuki beans are used in many other cuisines also, and can be found in supermarkets, natural food stores, and Asian markets throughout the United States. The Japanese boil adzuki beans with sugar to make a sweet red bean paste (*an*) that is used in desserts. Adzuki beans are also served with rice to make the

Asian version of rice and beans. Similar to soybeans, adzuki beans contain protease inhibitors that block enzymes that promote the growth of cancerous tumors. Adzuki beans are also an excellent source of fiber, which may protect against various forms of cancer as well as heart disease.

Bamboo Shoots Bamboo shoots are widely used in Asian cooking. They can be simmered in soups or sautéed in wok dishes with poultry, seafood, meat, or vegetables. They have a mild flavor and a crunchy texture. Canned shoots packed in water are available at Asian markets and supermarkets. Bamboo shoots are an excellent source of potassium, a mineral which helps regulate blood pressure and heart function.

Bean Sprouts Americans use croutons—often high in fat—to add crunch to a salad. In Asia, bean sprouts (usually mung bean) serve the same purpose, and are also used in many vegetable and stir-fry dishes. However, unlike croutons they are virtually calorie free, have no fat, and are a good source of vitamin C—a potent antioxidant that may protect against cancer and heart disease.

Bok Choy Also known in the United States as Chinese cabbage, bok choy is known as *hakusai* in Japan, and is popular among Asian chefs. In Japan, bok choy is often used in one-pot dishes such as sukiyaki, which include a mix of vegetables, noodles, and a small amount of meat. Bok choy is also sold in some supermarkets, greengrocers, and Asian markets in the United States. It may also be called celery cabbage or napa. Bok choy has a high amount of beta-carotene and vitamin C, two potent antioxidants that may protect against both cancer and heart disease. Bok choy is also a good source of calcium, a mineral that is essential for strong teeth and bones. A member of the cruciferous family, bok choy contains indoles—compounds which in animal studies have deactivated potent estrogens that can promote the growth of cancerous tumors.

Bonito, Dried For many centuries, bonito, a member of the mackerel family, has played an important role in Japanese cuisine. Packaged dried bonito flakes are sold in Asian markets. Dried bonito is an essential ingredient in *dashi,* Japanese soup stock. Shaved bonito pieces are often used as garnishes. Bonito is an excellent source of omega-3 fatty acids, which may protect against heart disease by lowering blood cholesterol and triglyceride levels, lowering blood pressure, and preventing the formation of tiny blood clots that could lodge in a coronary artery and cause a heart attack. Omega-3 fatty acids may also inhibit the growth of mammary tumors. (According to the National Heart and Lung Institute in the United States, just 1 gram of omega-3 fatty acids daily may reduce the risk of developing coronary artery disease by as much as 40 percent.)

Burdock The root of the burdock plant (*gobo*) has been used by traditional healers in both Japan and China for several centuries. In animal studies, extracts of burdock root have been shown to inhibit tumors. Burdock root should be washed well (it can be eaten skin and all) and stored in cold water to prevent discoloration. Burdock has a bland flavor that soaks up other flavors, and has a crunchy texture. Fresh burdock root is sold in Asian markets. Boiled, canned burdock is also available, but it is not as good as fresh.

Chrysanthemum (Leaves and Flower) In Japan, the dark green leaves of the chrysanthemum flower are commonly used in cooking. They may be parboiled and served in a salad, or added at the last minute to one-pot dishes such as sukiyaki. Green leafy vegetables in particular are abundant in beta-carotene, which may help prevent many different forms of cancer and heart disease. So judging by its bright green color, chrysanthemum leaves are probably a good source of beta-carotene, which converts to vitamin A in the body. In China, the chrysanthemum flower is made into a tea that is used externally to treat eye irritations and skin diseases. It is also drunk as a beverage to lower blood pressure. Dried chrysanthemum flowers are a symbol of longevity.

Daikon   Daikon is a white radish that grows longer than a foot and several inches thick. It is a common ingredient in Japanese cuisine. Grated daikon is used in tempura dipping sauce; thin-sliced daikon adds a crunchy texture to one-pot dishes or stews. Traditional Asian healers use daikon as a digestive aid. Daikon, as well as other members of the radish family, contain isothiniocyanates, which are believed to trigger the production of enzymes that protect against cancer. Daikon is sold in most Asian food stores and some greengrocers in the United States. Thin, raw slices of daikon are terrific dipped in a low-fat yogurt-based dressing.

Dashi   If you leaf through a Japanese cookbook, you will notice that many recipes call for *dashi,* much the same way an American cook book calls for chicken stock. *Dashi* is a soup stock that is made from dried bonito flakes (bonito is a member of the mackerel family) and kelp, a type of seaweed (see SEAWEED). You can make your own dashi by purchasing the ingredients at an Asian market, or you can buy dried, prepared *dashi.*

Eggplant   For most Americans, eggplant is a vegetable that you bread, fry, and douse with Parmesan cheese and tomato sauce. In Japanese cuisine, however, eggplant (*nasu*) is a very popular vegetable widely used in many dishes. Japanese eggplant is smaller, firmer, and sweeter than American eggplant. It is often grilled, simmered in one-pot dishes, or coated with batter and deep-fried for tempura. Eggplant is a member of the Solanaceae family, a group of vegetables being investigated by the National Cancer Institute for their potential cancer-fighting properties. Eggplant contains many important phytochemicals that may help to prevent cancer, including terpenes—antioxidants which may also deactivate the potent estrogens that contribute to tumor growth. Japanese eggplant is available in Asian markets. If you use American eggplants in Japanese recipes, use small eggplants.

Five Spice Powder A popular Chinese seasoning, five spice powder is a combination of five ground spices: star anise, anise pepper, fennel, cloves, and cinnamon. The seasoning is often used in cooking meat or poultry. Cinnamon, cloves, and fennel are good sources of chromium, a mineral which helps regulate blood sugar levels. In addition, spices such as these, which were at one time used as preservatives, are believed to contain antioxidants that may help prevent cancer and heart disease. Five spice powder is sold in Asian markets.

Ginger Known as *shoga* in Japanese, fresh ginger root is a common ingredient in Asian cooking. In fact, the Japanese often serve thin slices of pickled ginger between sushi courses to aid in digestion. Both Chinese and Japanese healers use ginger as a traditional herbal medicine. According to Ron Tee-guarden's *Chinese Tonic Herbs,* ginger "tones up the yang." (The Chinese believe that nature is divided into two opposing cycles, yin and yang. Yang represents action; yin represents the contemplative phase in which energy is restored.) In China, dried ginger is used to treat upset stomachs and to "warm up" the body. A tea brewed from ginger may help relieve cold symptoms. Ginger is on the list of foods being investigated by the National Cancer Institute for its potential anticancer properties. Studies show that ginger may inhibit the action of prostaglandin, which is responsible for triggering an inflammatory response in the body. Fresh ginger (never use powdered) is sold in Asian markets, greengrocers, and even in most supermarkets. Scrape off the brown peel before using it. Some recipes may call for juice and it is easy to make. Simply grate the fresh ginger, and squeeze in a cheesecloth bag into a bowl.

Ginkgo Nut The ginkgo tree is the oldest living tree on earth, dating back to pre–Ice Age times. For thousands of years, Asian healers have used the nut or kernel from the ginkgo tree to treat a wide range of medical problems. The meat of the ginkgo nut (*ginnan*) is a common ingredient in Japanese cooking, and can be grilled or used in stews or stir-fried dishes. The white nut turns green after cooking and has a pleasant, mild flavor. Fresh or canned ginkgo nuts (fresh have a much better flavor) are available in Asian markets and some natural food stores. Use a nutcracker to crack the outer thin beige shell. Inside, the nuts are covered by a brown skin. To loosen the skin, put the nuts in a pot of hot water over a low heat for a few minutes. Leave the nuts in the water and then gently peel the skin with a slotted spoon. In recent years, scientists have found that the leaf of the ginkgo tree contains potent antioxidants that may help protect against cancer and heart disease. Studies have also shown that extracts of the ginkgo leaf can improve the flow of blood throughout the body, especially to the brain. Ginkgo is being investigated as a treatment for Alzheimer's disease and asthma. In Europe, ginkgo extract is a leading over-the-counter drug taken to promote good circulation and improve memory. Although little research has been done on ginkgo nuts, it stands to reason that the fruit of this tree must contain some beneficial compounds.

Green Tea   If you've ever eaten at a Japanese restaurant, you have probably sipped a cup of green tea with your meal. The average Japanese person drinks several cups of green tea daily. Unfortunately, the average American rarely, if ever, drinks this healthful beverage. Unlike most teas sold in the United States, green tea is lightly processed and retains more important phytochemicals. Green tea is rich in compounds called *catechins* that, according to animal studies, can lower blood cholesterol levels, helping to prevent atherosclerosis. In addition, several studies have shown that the compounds in green tea can inhibit the growth of cancerous tumors. A recent study showed that green tea helped to slow the development of skin cancer in mice exposed to ultraviolet radiation. A cup of green tea daily may also help keep the dentist away. Studies show that compounds in green tea can kill bacteria in the mouth responsible for tooth decay. Green tea contains less than half the caffeine found in a cup of coffee.

Green tea is sold loose or in teabags in Asian food stores and most natural food stores.

Brewing Green Tea

Place 1 tablespoon of tea in a teaball and put it in 1 cup of boiling water. Let the mixture sit for 5 to 10 minutes. Remove the teaball and drink.

To make several cups at once, use a glass or ceramic teapot. Use 1 tablespoon of green tea for each cup of water. Pour boiling hot water over the tea, and let sit for about 10 minutes.

Harusame Noodles
These fine, white transparent noodles are made from potato flour and are terrific in a light vegetable soup or broth.

Hot Red Chili Pepper
Called *togarashi* in Japan, fresh or dried small red chili peppers are a popular seasoning in Asian cuisines. Chili peppers are high in beta-carotene and vitamin C, two potent antioxidants that may protect against cancer and heart disease. Capsaicin, a compound found in chili peppers, has been shown to lower both cholesterol and triglyceride levels in animals. Chili peppers can also help prevent the formation of dangerous blood clots that lead to a heart attack or stroke.

Kumquats
Kumquats are small, oval fruits in the citrus family. Kumquats have a distinctive tangy, sweet flavor. They are a good source of vitamin C.

Kudzu
Kudzu is used to thicken sauces and gravies throughout China and Japan. Made from the crushed, dried

root of the *Pueraria lobata* plant, kudzu has been used as a healing agent in Oriental medicine for more than 1,000 years. Oriental chefs prefer kudzu over Western thickening agents such as cornstarch because it creates a smooth, translucent sauce that looks as good as it feels in the mouth. It has a mild aroma and does not lump up or produce an uneven consistency. According to Chinese studies, kudzu is rich in flavonoids—compounds that help to strengthen and regulate capillaries or small blood vessels. Traditional healers use kudzu to relieve headaches, reduce high blood pressure, and treat alcoholism. In Japan, a tea made of kudzu root is used to treat allergies and asthma. (It's interesting to note that some of the newest and most effective medications for asthma are synthetic versions of flavonoids!) Kudzu is also used to soothe stomach distress and diarrhea. The powder is sold in natural food stores and Asian markets (sometimes called *arum root* powder). Kudzu comes in chunks of powder, and needs to be broken up and dissolved in a few tablespoons of cold water before it can be used in cooking.

Lemongrass Lemongrass, which is also called *citronella,* is a common ingredient in Thai and Vietnamese cooking and imparts a lemony flavor to food. Usually, the lower part of the stalk is crushed and finely chopped. Lemongrass is available at many Asian markets. Studies show that lemongrass oil may lower cholesterol. Researchers at the Department of Nutritional Sciences and Medicine at the University of Wisconsin gave men with high levels of blood cholesterol 140 milligrams of lemongrass oil daily for ninety days. Thirty-six percent of the men had a 10 percent drop in serum cholesterol.

Lichee Fruit Popular in China, this small, juicy fruit is often served as a dessert or used to sweeten poultry dishes. Lichee fruit can satisfy a sweet tooth without added calories or fat! (Dried lichees, which are a great snack, are called *lichee nuts.*) Lichees are sold in cans. Fresh lichees are available in the summer at Asian markets.

Licorice Root Licorice root is widely used in China in medicinal healing. Because of its sweet flavor, it is chewed like candy or made into tea. The compounds in licorice contain anti-inflammatory properties similar to cortisone; licorice is used as a treatment for ulcers, bowel disorders, and arthritis. A compound in licorice has been shown to kill the bacteria responsible for tooth decay. Researchers at the National Cancer Institute are investigating licorice for its potential as an anticancer drug. Licorice root or teas are available in Asian markets and natural food stores. Caution: Licorice should not be used by people who have high blood pressure.

Loquats This small, yellow fruit resembles an apricot. It is juicy and delicious and is often served for dessert after a Chinese meal. Try one and you won't even miss the typical Western high-sugar, fat-laden dessert.

Mirin Mirin is a sweet wine made from fermented rice. It offsets the salty taste of soy sauce, and is frequently used in noodle and meat dishes. In Japan, a drink made from mirin and medicinal herbs is used to toast the New Year. Mirin is sold in Asian markets.

Onions Many Asian recipes call for some form of onion, a member of the allium family. The Japanese use *aoenegi,* a long, green onion, or *rakkyo,* a type of shallot. Chinese chefs typically use scallions and yellow onions. An old folk remedy for a variety of ailments, onions are being investigated by the National Cancer Institute for their potential cancer-fighting properties. In addition, studies show that onions can help reduce blood cholesterol levels, lower blood pressure, and prevent dangerous blood clots. A 1989 Chinese study described in the *Journal of the National Cancer Institute* showed that people who ate the highest amounts of onion had the lowest rates of stomach cancer.

Persimmon Known as *kaki* in Japan, persimmon fruit is often served as dessert. It has a sweet, slightly spicy flavor and goes well with the spices used in Japanese cooking. Fresh persimmon is available from September to November. It is a good source of fiber and potassium.

Red Jujube Dates

Used in Chinese cooking, these small, dried red dates with wrinkled skins are added to soups, stews, meat, and poultry dishes as a sweetener. Since ancient times they have been used by Chinese herbalists to lower blood pressure, improve heart function, and serve as a mild sedative. A "yin" herb, jujube is often used along with ginseng, a "yang" herb that energizes the body. Red jujube dates are sold in many Asian markets.

Reishi Mushrooms

Known as *kisshotake* or the "lucky fungus," in Japan, reishi mushrooms were originally used in China in both cooking and traditional healing. However, for several thousand years the Japanese have used these delicately flavored mushrooms in their cuisine. Reishi mushrooms, which are quite pricey, are available in Asian markets and gourmet shops. However, they may be worth their weight in gold. Recent studies show that reishi may stimulate the immune system, which increases the body's ability to ward off disease. In addition, reishi mushrooms contain compounds that are natural antihistamines and have strong anti-allergic activity. Other studies show that reishi can lower blood cholesterol levels and prevent the formation of dangerous blood clots that can lead to a heart attack or stroke.

Seaweed

The average per capita intake of seaweed in Japan ranges from 4.9 to 7.0 grams daily, but few Americans eat this food. Dietary seaweed is sold in the United States in Asian and natural food stores. There are several varieties of seaweed or algae, differentiated by their color. *Nori,* a red seaweed, is used to wrap sushi. (When dried, it takes on a dark green color.) Popular forms of brown seaweed include kelp, *wakame, arme,* and *kombu.*

Traditional Chinese healers have used hot water extracts of seaweed to treat cancer. Recent studies show that compounds in seaweed may protect against cancer. Japanese scientists isolated several polysaccharides, potentially anticarcinogenic compounds in seaweed. Fucoidin, one of these compounds, may prove to be a potent cancer fighter. Researchers speculate that the seaweed may somehow boost the body's immunological defenses against tumor growth. However, test-tube studies also show that seaweed extract can prevent or slow down the growth of cancer cells outside the body, which suggests that it may also inhibit the growth of cells on its own.

Studies show that seaweed also helps reduce cholesterol levels, and may help rid the body of toxic metals.

Nori can be eaten right out of the package (it comes in a flat roll), or can be used as a seasoning in stews. *Wakame* is good in salads.

Sesame Oil and Seeds

Oriental sesame oil is frequently used as a flavoring in Japanese and Chinese cooking. (It burns very easily, so it is not usually used in cooking.) Toasted black or white sesame seeds are often used as a condiment to add crunch and a delicate, nutty flavor to foods. Studies suggest that sesame may protect against both cancer and heart disease. In one Japanese study published in the *Japanese Journal of Cancer Research,* sesame oil reduced the amount of bile acids in the feces of rats. Bile acids are believed to produce cancerous changes in the cells of the intestinal wall, which may cause colon cancer. Thus, by reducing the amount of bile, sesame may protect against colon cancer. Sesame seeds are also an excellent source of phytic acid, an antioxidant that is also present in soy. In another study, researchers injected various spice extracts into mice with tumors. Although all the spices increased the life span of the mice, only the sesame extract produced any significant reduction in tumor growth. In a study that appeared in the *Journal of Lipid Research,* sesamin, a lignin from sesame oil, was fed to rats to investigate its effect on cholesterol metabolism. Sesamin significantly reduced the amount of serum and liver cholesterol in rats fed a normal diet. (However, when the rats were fed a diet entirely free of cholesterol, the sesamin had no effect.) Based on this study, researchers speculate that sesamin may be a useful cholesterol lowering agent.

Seven Spice Powder
Known as *shichimi* in Japan, this widely used seasoning contains a mixture of seven spices: chili pepper, black pepper, ground orange peel, sesame seeds, poppy seeds, hemp seeds, and powdered *nori* (seaweed). Several of these ingredients offer potential health benefits. Chili protects against cardiovascular disease (see HOT RED CHILI PEPPER). Orange peel contains citrus oils, which may inhibit the growth of tumors. Poppy seeds are a good source of chromium, a mineral which helps regulate blood sugar levels. Hemp seeds are used by Asian healers to treat a variety of ailments. And *nori* may help protect against cancer (see SEAWEED). Seven spice powder is sold at Asian markets.

Shark Fin
In China, the dried cartilage of the shark fin is considered a delicacy. It is often served in a thick soup at banquets and on special occasions. Cartilage is a good source of protein and calcium. In recent years, shark cartilage has garnered much publicity, largely owing to the book *Sharks Don't Get Cancer,* which touts shark cartilage as a potent cancer fighter. Dried shark fin cartilage is sold in Asian food stores—it is very expensive. It must be soaked overnight in warm water before it can be used in cooking.

Shiitake Mushrooms
Shiitake mushrooms, grown in the forests of Japan and in the United States, are a common ingredient in Japanese cooking. Fresh or dried shiitake mushrooms are available in Asian food stores or greengrocers. Shiitake is highly revered in the Orient for its potential health benefits. Several studies show that shiitake can lower blood cholesterol, thus helping protect against heart disease. In addition, shiitake contains a compound called lentinen, which can stimulate the immune system to ward off infections and viruses. In Japan, lentinen is used as a treatment for cancer. Researchers at the Yamaguchi University School of Medicine

in Japan are investigating shiitake as a potential cancer treatment.

Shirataki   These long, white noodles are made from yams. They are used in sukiyaki and other one-pot dishes. They are very low in calories and are fat free.

Soba   Soba noodles, which are a major ingredient in Japanese cuisine, are made from buckwheat, the fruit of the *Pagopyrum* genus, which is related to rhubarb. Dried soba noodles can be found in Asian markets and natural food stores. Similar to soybeans, buckwheat is one of the few plant foods that is abundant in lysine, an essential amino acid usually found in foods of animal origin. Buckwheat also contains a bioflavonoid called *rutin*, which is used to treat capillary fragility, a condition characterized by easy bruising and bleeding gums. Studies show that buckwheat may also help to keep glucose levels under control more efficiently than other types of carbohydrates, which makes it a good food choice for diabetics.

Spinach   Known as *horenso,* Japanese spinach is sweeter and milder tasting than the Western variety. The leaves are smaller and more delicate. Horenso is sold with the pink roots attached, which can be eaten. Japanese spinach is available in Asian markets.

Udon Noodles   These thick wheat noodles, usually made from whole wheat or a combination of whole wheat and unbleached white wheat, are excellent in soups. Whole wheat is a good source of fiber, B vitamins, and potassium. Similar to linguine, udon noodles hold the sauce well. They are available at Asian markets. Udon noodles made from brown rice are sold in natural food stores.

Wasabi   Wasabi is a condiment made from the *Wasabia japonica* plant. Similar to Western horseradish, it usually is served with sushi (raw fish). Fresh wasabi root is hard to find in the United States, but wasabi powder or paste is sold in most Asian markets.

Ten

Earl's Pearls: A Guide to Vitamins and Minerals

No man or woman can live by soy alone. Vitamins and minerals play a critical role in maintaining health. Here's a list of the major players, what they do, and where to find them.

*   *   *

Know Your Vitamins

A *Stands for Beta-carotene* . . .

Vitamin A is known as the skin vitamin because it is essential for healthy skin and mucous membranes. It is essential for the normal functioning of the immune system. Synthetic forms of vitamin A are used to treat acne, psoriasis, and even some skin cancers.

Pure vitamin A, known as preformed vitamin A, can be toxic at doses over 5,000 milligrams daily. However, beta-carotene (also called provitamin A), a compound found in food plants, can be converted into vitamin A as the body needs it. There is no evidence that beta-carotene is toxic at any dose. Beta-carotene is a potent antioxidant; vitamin A is not. Numerous studies suggest that beta-carotene may protect against many different forms of cancer, including oral cancers, stomach cancer, bladder cancer, breast cancer, and cervical cancer. Recent studies also suggest that beta-carotene may help protect against atherosclerosis by preventing the oxidation of LDL, or "bad cholesterol." Beta-carotene may also help strengthen the immune function in people with HIV.

Good food sources of beta-carotene include dark leafy vegetables and yellow and orange fruits and vegetables. Bok choy (see Chapter 9) is brimming with beta-carotene!

The RDA for vitamin A is 5,000 International Units (IU) or 1,000 Retinol Equivalent (RE). Doses over 25,000 IU of vitamin A can be toxic. Vitamin A can cause birth defects, and should not be taken by pregnant women. The RDA for beta-carotene is 3 milligrams which equals 5,000 IU vitamin A. However, many researchers feel that people need about 6 milligrams of beta-carotene daily.

Getting to Know the B-Complex Family

B₁ (Thiamine) B_1 breaks down and converts carbohydrates into glucose, which provides energy for the body. B_1 is necessary for the normal functioning of the nervous system, heart, and other muscles. Deficiency of this B vitamin can result in depression, lethargy, loss of appetite, and numbness in the legs. In times of stress, you may need more of B_1 and other B vitamins. Good food sources of thiamine include brewer's yeast, rice husks, unrefined cereal grains, sunflower seeds, pecans, lean pork, green peas, most vegetables, and milk. The RDA for thiamine for adults is 1.0 to 1.5 milligrams. Thiamine can be destroyed by alcohol; alcoholics and heavy drinkers are at risk of thiamine deficiency. Thiamine is usually included in B-complex supplements and multivitamins.

B₂ (Riboflavin) This B vitamin works with other substances to metabolize carbohydrates, fats, and proteins for energy. Riboflavin may also protect against certain forms of cancer and the oxidative damage of free radicals.

Good sources of riboflavin include nonfat or low-fat dairy products, reduced-fat soy milk, eggs, and leafy vegetables. The RDA is 1.2 to 1.7 milligrams for adults. Riboflavin is included in most multivitamin supplements, as well as in B-complex supplements. The usual dose is 100 to 300 milligrams. Women who take estrogen need to take a B_1 supplement.

Riboflavin works best with vitamins B_6, C, and niacin. A particularly important role of riboflavin is to protect against oxidative damage during exercise, when the demand for oxygen by the body increases. Riboflavin can help to prevent damage to the cornea of the eye, such as cataracts. Riboflavin deficiency can decrease the number of T-cells, an important component of the immune system. Low levels of T-cells may increase the risk of developing cancer and other diseases.

B₃ (Niacin) Vitamin B_3 works with B_1 and B_2 to metabolize carbohydrates and is essential for providing energy for cell tissue growth. Niacin is necessary for a healthy nervous system and normal brain function. Taken as a supplement, B_3 has been shown to significantly cut blood cholesterol and blood triglyceride levels, working as well as many of the cholesterol-lowering drugs. Good food sources include mackerel, swordfish, chicken, and fortified cereals. The RDA for niacin is 13 to 19 milligrams for adults, and 20 milligrams for nursing mothers. High doses of niacin can trigger diabetes in people with prediabetic conditions, and can also bring about attacks of gout for people prone to that disease and can cause liver damage. High doses of niacin can also cause temporary flushing or itching, which can be quite uncomfortable; niacinamide and nicotinamide, two forms of niacin, do not cause flushing. (For information on how niacin can be used safely and comfortably to lower cholesterol, see Chapter 4.)

B_6 (Pyridoxine)

Vitamin B_6 helps the body properly assimilate protein and fat to build body tissue. It is also essential in the formation of nucleic acid, which is needed to replace old and dying cells. Even a mild B_6 deficiency can hamper the normal functioning of the immune system. A recent study showed that people with the lowest blood levels of B_6 (and folic acid, another B vitamin) had the highest blood levels of homocysteine in the blood, a possible risk factor for heart attack. Good food sources of B_6 include soybeans, brewer's yeast, fortified ready-to-eat cereals, and chicken. The RDA for B_6 is 1.6 milligrams for adult women and 2 milligrams for adult men.

B_{12} (Cobalamin)

Known as the "red vitamin," B_{12} aids in the formation of red blood cells, in the normal functioning of the nervous system, and in the metabolism of protein and fat. Folic acid, another B vitamin, cannot be properly utilized by the body without B_{12}. Vitamin B_{12} deficiency can result in pernicious anemia. Even a mild B_{12} deficiency in older people can result in confusion, weakness, and memory loss that is often confused with senility or Alzheimer's disease. Good food sources of B_{12} include meat, fish, eggs, dairy products, and fortified soy milk. Tempeh (made from fermented soybeans) is one of the few food plants that is rich in B_{12}. Vegetarians beware: you may not be getting enough B_{12}. The RDA for B_{12} is 2 micrograms for both men and women.

Biotin   This B vitamin is essential for the metabolism of fat and protein and for the absorption of vitamin C. Biotin is important for healthy skin. Good food sources include brewer's yeast, fruit, nuts, peanut butter, and whole-grain foods. The RDA for biotin is 300 micrograms.

Folic Acid (Folacin)   Folic acid helps in the formation of red blood cells and genetic material in the cells. A deficiency of this vitamin during pregnancy increases the risk of having a child with neural tube defects. Folic acid may also protect against colon and rectal cancer and cancer of the cervix. Good food sources of folic acid include dark green leafy vegetables, liver, and fortified grains. Legumes such as soybeans are also high in folic acid. The RDA for folic acid is 400 micrograms. Caution: People taking anticonvulsive medications should check with their physicians before taking folic acid.

Pantothenic Acid   This B vitamin helps convert nutrients into energy. Recent studies show that pantothenic acid supplements can lower cholesterol and triglycerides. Good food sources include legumes such as soybeans, peanuts, wheat germ, and lean meats. The RDA for pantothenic acid is 10 milligrams. People who are on a cholesterol-lowering program may be given doses as high as 1,000 milligrams daily by their physicians.

Vitamin C—Linus Pauling was Right!

Vitamin C is the most popular vitamin supplement in the country and for good reason. More than two decades ago, Nobel laureate Linus Pauling suggested that this vitamin may play a special role in the prevention and treatment of disease.

Recent studies show that he was right. Vitamin C (also called *ascorbic acid*) is necessary for the formation of collagen, which is essential for the growth and repair of all body cells. Vitamin C can lessen severity and duration of the common cold. Vitamin C is an antioxidant—it protects body cells from destruction by free radicals. It also deactivates carcinogens that may promote cancer. In fact, several studies suggest that vitamin C may help protect against many different forms of cancer, including oral cancers, lung cancer, breast cancer, stomach cancer, bladder cancer, and pancreatic cancer. Vitamin C may also help to ward off heart disease by preventing the oxidation of LDL, or "bad cholesterol," which can lead to the formation of atherosclerotic lesions or plaque. Good food sources of vitamin C include sweet red pepper, broccoli, orange juice, tomatoes, and berries. The RDA for vitamin C is 60 milligrams. I feel that people need to take 1,000 to 2,000 milligrams of vitamin C daily. (Calcium ascorbate is the best form of vitamin C—it's gentlest on your stomach.)

Vitamin D: Let a Little Sunshine into Your Life

Ultraviolet rays from the sun stimulate oils in the skin to produce vitamin D, which works with calcium and phosphorus to produce strong teeth and bones. Studies show that in climates where there is little sunshine (and less vitamin D is produced by the body), there are higher rates of colon cancer. In addition, in a recent study, vitamin D and calcium were shown to reduce winter bone loss in women, which could reduce the risk of getting osteoporosis. (Because of reduced activity owing to cold weather and less exposure to sun, bone loss accelerates during winter months.) Good food sources of vitamin D include fatty fish (mackerel, salmon, and sardines) and fortified dairy products. The RDA for vitamin D is 400 IU. Very large doses of vitamin D over a long period of time can be toxic.

Vitamin E: Superstar Among Vitamins

Vitamin E—once maligned as a "do-nothing vitamin" by the medical establishment—is now championed by some of the biggest names in medicine. Also known as tocopherol, vitamin E is a potent antioxidant that may protect against cancer, heart disease, and premature aging. In a recent study of 40,000 male medical professionals, those taking a vitamin E supplement had a 40 percent lower risk of developing heart disease. A study among women yielded similar results. A study at the Johns Hopkins School of Hygiene and Public Health showed that people with the lowest blood serum levels of vitamin E had the highest risk of developing lung cancer. Vitamin E is synergistic with a mineral, selenium, which means they enhance each other's action. Vitamin E also appears to boost immune function. Good food sources of vitamin E include vegetable oils, whole grains, wheat germ, brown rice, oatmeal, and nuts. The RDA for vitamin E is 8 to 10 IU. I recommend taking 400 IU of vitamin E daily.

Vitamin K—For Blood and Bones

This vitamin is essential for proper blood clotting. Recent studies suggest that it is also important for calcium absorption, which means that it may play an indirect role in helping prevent osteoporosis. Good food sources of vitamin K include soybean oil, green leafy vegetables, broccoli, alfalfa, cooked spinach, and fish oils. The RDA for vitamin K is 65 to 80 micrograms. Doses over 500 micrograms daily can be dangerous. Do not take a vitamin K supplement if you are taking a blood thinner.

The Minerals of Life

Boron for Bones

Boron, a mineral found in fruits and vegetables, appears to work with calcium and magnesium to build strong bones. Boron increases blood serum levels of estrogen in women, and estrogen helps retain calcium and magnesium. Good food sources of boron include dried fruits. There is no RDA for boron. I recommend 3 milligrams daily.

Calcium for Just About Everything

Calcium is used for building strong teeth and bones and in keeping them strong and healthy. It is also important for maintenance of cell membranes, blood clotting, and muscle absorption. Calcium can help lower blood pressure in people with high blood pressure and may also play a role in keeping cholesterol levels in check. A calcium deficiency may increase the risk of developing colon cancer. Calcium supplements are often prescribed as a treatment for premenstrual syndrome (PMS). Good sources of calcium are low-fat or nonfat dairy products, kale, tofu made with calcium sulfate, broccoli, canned salmon or sardines with bones, and calcium-fortified fruit juice. The RDA for adults up to twenty-five years is 1,200 milligrams, and from twenty-five to fifty, 800 milligrams. Most women and younger men consume less than half the calcium they need. Postmenopausal women should get 1,500 milligrams of calcium daily, but few do.

Vitamin D helps facilitate calcium absorption.

Chromium for Normal Blood Sugar

Chromium works with insulin in the metabolism of sugar. Chromium has also been used to raise HDL, or "good cholesterol," in diabetics. Chromium picolinate, a better absorbed form of chromium, can lower cholesterol in people with mildly elevated cholesterol levels. Good food sources of chromium include broccoli, brewer's yeast, and shellfish. There is no RDA for chromium. For adults, I recommend 50 to 200 micrograms daily.

Copper for Your Blood, Joints, and Heart

Copper is necessary to convert iron into hemoglobin, the substance that gives red blood cells their color. Copper may also help play a role in dissolving blood clots in the body. If a blood clot lodges in an artery leading to the heart or the brain, it could cause a heart attack or stroke. Copper may also help to reduce the inflammation caused by arthritis. In fact, copper is included in many arthritis medications. Good food sources include legumes such as soybeans, whole wheat, nuts, and seeds. There is no RDA for copper. The National Academy of Sciences' Estimated Safe and Adequate Dietary Intake is between 1.5 and 3 milligrams daily.

Fluoride for Teeth and Bones

Fluoride is added to the drinking water in many communities because it can help to prevent tooth decay. Recent studies suggest that people who live in areas with fluoridated water have a lower risk of developing osteoporosis. Good food sources are seafood, gelatin, and fluoridated drinking water. There is no RDA. The National Academy of Sciences' Estimated

Safe and Adequate Dietary Intake is between 1.5 and 4 milligrams.

Iodine for Your Thyroid

Iodine is essential for the normal functioning of the thyroid gland An iodine deficiency can lead to a sluggish thyroid, which can result in fatigue, weight gain, and puffiness under the chin. Good food sources include iodized salt, seaweed, onions, and seafood. The RDA is 150 micrograms for adults.

Iron for Blood

Iron is a blood builder: it is necessary for the production of hemoglobin, red blood corpuscles, and myoglobin—all important components of healthy blood. A deficiency in this mineral can lead to iron deficiency anemia, characterized by fatigue and always feeling cold. Women with heavy menstrual periods are prone to iron deficiency anemia. Good food sources include meat and poultry, however soybeans (and other legumes), dried fruit, and green vegetables also contain iron. Iron is best utilized when taken with vitamin C. The RDA is 15 milligrams for premenopausal women; 10 milligrams for postmenopausal women and men. Excess iron intake has been linked to heart disease. If you take supplemental iron, be sure to take it with an antioxidant.

Magnesium for Heart and Bones

Magnesium works with other minerals to build strong bones, manufacture proteins, and regulate heartbeat and muscle contraction. Studies show that magnesium can lower blood pressure, relieve migraine headaches, and improve glucose handling in older people. (As people age, they become less efficient in their use of insulin, which can result in insulin resistance.) Good food sources include bananas, apricots, curry powder, wheat bran, and whole grains. The RDA for adults is 250 to 350 milligrams daily. Pregnant women need 300 to 355 milligrams daily.

Manganese: An Important Helper

Few people worry about getting enough manganese, and yet this mineral performs many important jobs in the body. Manganese activates the enzymes that are necessary for the utilization of biotin, vitamin B_1, and vitamin C. It is needed to form strong bones, and may play a role in preventing osteoporosis. Manganese is also essential for the proper functioning of the production of sex hormones and the proper functioning of the nervous system. Manganese is an antioxidant. Good food sources include green leafy vegetables, nuts, peas, whole grains, and egg yolks. There is no RDA, but most adults should get between 2.5 and 5 milligrams of this mineral.

Molybdenum for Metabolism

You probably never heard of this mineral, but it is important because it aids in carbohydrate and fat metabolism. It is also necessary for the proper utilization of iron. Molybdenum is present in whole grains, green leafy vegetables, and legumes such as soybeans. Supplementation is rarely necessary. There is no RDA but the estimated daily intake should be around 75 to 250 micrograms.

Phosphorus: Calcium's Helper

Phosphorus works with calcium to build strong teeth and bones. Phosphorus is involved in nearly every important chemical reaction in the body. Phosphorus is found in many foods, including fish, poultry, meat, whole grains, eggs, nuts, and seeds. The RDA is 800 milligrams for adults, 1,200 milligrams for pregnant and lactating women.

Potassium for Normal Blood Pressure

This mineral helps to regulate the body's water balance and normalize heart rhythm. A recent study showed that an increase in dietary potassium can significantly reduce blood pressure in hypertensive people. In fact, many people were able to reduce or even discontinue their medication simply by eating potassium-rich foods. Low intake of potassium can result in an irregular heartbeat. Potassium is also essential for the normal functioning of nerves and muscles. Good food sources of potassium include white potatoes, dried apricots, lima beans, orange juice, prunes, and sweet potatoes. There is no RDA. The National Academy of Sciences' Estimated Safe and Adequate Daily Dietary Intake for potassium is 1,600 to 2,000 milligrams daily. People with kidney problems should avoid potassium-rich foods and should not take potassium supplements.

Selenium for Cancer and Stroke Prevention

This mineral works with glutathione, a tripeptide in the body. It is also synergistic with vitamin E, meaning that the combination of the two is far more potent than either one alone. Selenium is an antioxidant: it protects cells against damage inflicted by free radicals or unstable molecules that can damage DNA and trigger cancerous growths. People who live in areas where the soil is rich in selenium (and therefore is present in the locally grown food and water) have significantly lower incidence of stroke than do people who live in selenium-poor areas. Good food sources of selenium include broccoli, garlic, whole wheat, onions, and red grapes. The RDA is 50 to 100 micrograms daily. Many cancer researchers feel that 200 micrograms of selenium are necessary to protect against cancer. Doses over 200 micrograms may be toxic.

Sodium for Balance

Sodium works with potassium to help the body maintain a normal fluid balance. Too much sodium can cause high blood pressure in salt-sensitive individuals. (Most people excrete excess salt in urine, however some people may retain salt and excess fluid. The body must work harder to pump excess fluid, resulting in a rise in blood pressure.) Sodium is found in table salt and occurs naturally in food, and is often added to processed foods. The American Heart Association recommends that you limit your sodium intake to 2,400 milligrams daily.

Zinc for Healing, Prostate, and the Common Cold

Zinc is involved in cell division, growth, and repair. It is essential for wound healing. High concentrations of zinc are found in the male prostate gland, and a shortage of this mineral may play a role in male infertility. (Oysters, which are high in zinc, have been touted as aphrodisiac for years!) Recent studies suggest that zinc lozenges (available in natural food stores) may protect against the common cold. Good food sources include soybeans and other legumes, brewer's yeast, lamb chops, eggs, liver, wheat germ, and pumpkin seeds.

Other Cancer Fighters

Astralagus

Native to China and Japan, this herb is an immune booster that may help the body's own defense system against cancer. Researchers at the University of Texas Medical Center in Houston found that a purified extract of astralagus stimulates T-cells (one of the key white cells of the immune system) in healthy animals and helps normalize the immune systems of cancer patients with impaired immunity owing to chemotherapy. Other studies have shown that astralagus can stimulate the production of interferon, a protein produced in cells that fights against viral invasion.

Beta-carotene

Beta-carotene is a naturally occurring compound found in green and yellow fruits and vegetables. Beta-carotene, a potent antioxidant, is converted to vitamin A as the body needs it. Numerous studies have shown that beta-carotene may protect against many different forms of cancer including lung cancer, breast cancer, cervical cancer, colorectal cancer, bladder cancer, and oral cancers.

Catechins

Catechins are compounds found in tea, berries, and other fruits and vegetables that can inhibit the growth of cancerous tumors. (Japanese green tea is an excellent source of catechins.)

D-limonene

Limonene, a compound found in orange and lemon peels, can inhibit the growth of breast cancer cells in animals. A recent study performed at Duke Medical Center showed that high doses of limonene increases the production of the protein TGF-beta, which programs breast cancer cells in rats to self-destruct. Limonene belongs to a group of compounds called *monoterpenes* that are being investigated by the National Cancer Institute for their potential anticancer activity.

Ellagic acid

Ellagic acid is a polyphenolic compound found in strawberries, cherries, and grapes. Animal studies show that ellagic acid counteracts synthetic and naturally occurring carcinogens, thus preventing healthy cells form turning cancerous. Ellagic acid is also an antioxidant that may block the destructive effects of free radicals. Ellagic acid's ability to counteract carcinogens is very promising. For example, in a Japanese study, laboratory rats were fed a diet high in various polyphenol compounds. One group was given ellagic acid exclusively. The rats were later exposed to a potent carcinogen to induce tongue cancer. All of the rats on the various polyphenolic compounds had a reduced incidence of cancer, however those on the ellagic acid remained entirely cancer free. The researchers speculated that ellagic acid (and other polyphenols) may help to prevent cancer in other tissues, including skin, lung, liver, and the esophagus

Indoles

These compounds, found in broccoli and other cruciferous vegetables, may inactivate potent estrogens that can stimulate the growth of tumors in estrogen-sensitive cells.

Lignans

Lignans are a form of fiber found in grains, seeds, and legumes. Flax is abundant in lignans; among commonly used grains, however, rye is one of the best sources. Similar to the isoflavones found in soy, lignans are converted by gut bacteria to estrogenlike compounds that may also bind to estrogen receptors and "down regulate" estrogen. Thus, lignans may also protect against hormone-dependent cancers. Research has shown that women who consume high amounts of lignans have lower levels of breast cancer and colon cancer.

Lycopene

Found in red pepper, ruby red grapefruits, and tomato, this member of the carotene family is an antioxidant. Recent studies suggest that it may protect against cervical cancer.

Omega-3 Fatty Acids

Found in fatty fish, soy oil, and purslane (a weed that has become a popular salad ingredient), omega-3 fatty acids tested in animal studies have shown that they can shrink mammary tumors.

Pectin

A form of soluble fiber found in food plants, pectin may bind with bile acids and possibly toxins in the intestine, flushing them out of the system via the feces. High levels of bile acids and exposure to certain toxins in the gut are believed to promote colon cancer.

Quercetin

Quercetin, a bioflavonoid, is found in yellow and red onions and shallots, broccoli, and Italian squash. In many studies, quercetin has been shown to block the action of a variety of natural and synthetic initiators or promoters of cancer-cell development. In addition, quercetin appears to inhibit the growth of human tumor cells containing binding sites for type-II estrogen, which may be responsible for some forms of cancer, including breast cancer.

Retinoids

Retinoids are a related family of compounds (including vitamin A) that may offer protection against lung and oral cancers. A potent synthetic form of vitamin A is used as a treatment for skin cancer.

Sulfides

Found in garlic and onions, these compounds have been shown in animal studies to deactivate potent carcinogens. One type of sulfide found in garlic, diallyl, has been shown to reduce the metabolism of nitrosamine (a potent naturally occurring carcinogen) by the liver.

Sulforaphane

A compound found in cruciferous vegetables (cabbage, broccoli, kale, Brussels sprouts), sulforaphane stimulates animal and human cells to produce cancer-fighting enzymes.

Wheat bran

Researchers at the American Health Foundation tested various types of fiber to see which, if any, could reduce the level of potent estrogens in women. For two months premenopausal women had their diets supplemented with 30 grams of either wheat bran, corn bran, or oat bran. Only the wheat bran could significantly reduce the level of estrone and estradiol, two potent estrogens that could promote the growth of tumors in estrogen-sensitive cells.

More Cholesterol Busters

As good as soy may be as a cholesterol-lowering agent, there are other natural substances that can give you a winning edge in the battle of the blood lipids.

- *Alfalfa sprouts*—Studies show that alfalfa sprouts lower cholesterol in people with high cholesterol. (People with lupus should avoid alfalfa sprouts.)

- *Apple*—Apple is an excellent source of pectin, a type of soluble fiber that seems to melt cholesterol away, especially LDL, or "bad" cholesterol.

- *Carrots*—Carrots are a good source of calcium pectate, a form of fiber that lowers cholesterol.

- *Chili peppers*—Capsaicin, a compound found in hot chili peppers, reduces cholesterol and triglycerides.

- *Chromium*—Animal studies show that this mineral can lower cholesterol and raise HDL. I recommend chromium picolinate, a better absorbed form of chromium. Take 200 micrograms daily. (See NIACIN.)

- *Curry*—The spices in curry powder contain chromium and antioxidants that help to lower cholesterol.

- *Eggplant*—Studies show that eggplant helps lower the amount of cholesterol absorbed from fatty foods.

- *Fiber*—Fiber, the indigestible compounds found in food plants, helps to lower blood cholesterol levels. Soluble fiber, such as pectin and plant gums (such as guar gum), are particularly potent cholesterol busters.

- *Garlic*—Several studies show that garlic can lower cholesterol in animals and humans. An added bonus: garlic contains a compound called *ajoene,* which also helps to prevent blood clots.

- *Grapefruit*—The pulpy membrane in grapefruit is rich in pectin, which lowers cholesterol.

- *Green tea*—Popular in Japan, green tea contains catechins, which have lowered cholesterol in animal studies.

- *Legumes*—Dried beans including lentils, black beans, and navy beans have been shown to lower cholesterol in people with high cholesterol.

- *Niacin*—Vitamin B$_3$, also known as niacin, is an excellent cholesterol-lowering agent that also raises HDL. In high doses, niacin can cause flushing, headache, itching, and liver damage. I recommend no-flush niacin supplements with inositol hexanicotinate, which may relieve some of the discomfort. I also recommend a chromium-niacin supplement (200 micrograms of chromium bound to 2 milligrams niacin). These two compounds are synergistic—that is, the two combined are far more powerful than either one separately. Niacin should not be used by borderline diabetics or people with gout. People taking niacin to lower cholesterol should be monitored by their physicians.

- *Oat bran*—If you have high cholesterol, oat bran can help bring it down by as much as 12 percent.

- *Olive oil*—Olive oil is rich in monounsaturated fats. Although it may not reduce total cholesterol, it does raise the level of HDLs, the so-called good cholesterol.

- *Omega-3 fatty acids*—Found primarily in fatty fish such as mackerel, salmon, and albacore tuna, omega-3 fatty acids can reduce cholesterol and triglycerides in people with high cholesterol.

- *Onion*—Studies show that people who eat onions can raise their HDL, or "good" cholesterol.

- *Psyllium*—Used in many bulk laxatives and added to some cereals, psyllium is rich in soluble fiber. Studies show that it can significantly lower cholesterol among people with high cholesterol and, in particular, lower the level of LDL.

- *Red wine*—Red wine contains resveratol, which has been shown to lower cholesterol in animals. Human studies have shown that moderate wine drinkers have lower cholesterol, higher HDL, and a reduced risk of heart disease.

Part IV

GET MORE SOY
IN YOUR LIFE!

Eleven

Savvy
Substitutions

S oy foods can be used to replace meat and dairy products
in a variety of ways. Here are just some examples of how
you can get more soy into your life!

Baked Goods

Soy Flour

- Substitute up to 20 percent of soy flour in recipes calling for flour. (Soy flour does not contain gluten, there-

fore, it cannot be used as the sole flour in yeast-raised products.)

•　In recipes that are not yeast raised, you can substitute up to 25 percent of the total flour with soy flour. (If a recipe is specially designed for soy flour, you can use more.)

•　Soy flour can be used to thicken gravies and cream sauces.

•　If you're frying foods such as doughnuts, using soy flour can reduce the amount of fat absorbed by the food.

Isolated Soy Protein

Isolated soy protein (ISP) added to baked goods offers a protein boost as well as some of the beneficial compounds found in soy, such as isoflavones and phytic acid. In addition, ISP can help lower cholesterol.

Dairy

Soy Milk

Soy milk can be used as a nondairy, lactose-free, cholesterol-free substitute in just about any recipe that calls for cow's milk.

•　Drink a glass of ice-cold soy milk instead of dairy milk for a low-fat, cholesterol-free alternative. Soy milk comes plain and flavored, including malt, chocolate, strawberry, and my favorite, Westbrae 1% Lite vanilla.

•　Pour soy milk over cold or hot cereal.

•　Use soy milk to make a terrific pudding.

•　Use soy milk instead of cream when cooking—you get the creamy, rich texture of real cream, but without the real fat!

- Replace evaporated milk with soy milk for a luscious pie filling or custard. (Try the Chocolate Cream Pie on page 221.)

- Whip up a "milk" shake in your blender using soy milk and fresh fruit.

Tofu

Tofu's creamy, cheeselike texture makes it a natural dairy substitute in recipes calling for milk, cream, or cheese.

- Try tofu as a topping for pizza or as a cheese substitute in lasagna. When melted and mixed with tomato sauce and Italian seasoning, it's difficult to tell the difference between tofu and real cheese.

- Tofu makes a wonderful low-fat base for cream soups.

- Blended tofu with vegetables or spices makes a delicious "cream cheese" or dip.

- Mixed with fruit and other flavors, tofu can be made into a delicious low-fat frozen dessert.

Prepared Soy "Dairy" Products

There is a wide selection of prepared nondairy soy products geared primarily for people who want or need to avoid dairy. Some of these products include soy yogurt, soy frozen desserts, and a variety of soy imitation cheese and spreads. In most cases these products can substitute for dairy products in cooking. There are even some prepared foods, such as pizza or "cheese" enchiladas that use tofu instead of cheese. Check the dairy counter of your local supermarket or natural food stores.

Eggs

Soy Flour

- To replace eggs in baked goods, use 1 tablespoon of soy flour and 1 tablespoon of water per egg.

- For cholesterol watchers, tofu can replace eggs in a recipe. Use 1 ounce mashed tofu for every egg.

Tofu

- Tofu can be "scrambled" with spices and vegetables for a cholesterol-free omelette.

- Diced tofu can be mixed with celery, onions, light mayonnaise, and spices for a delicious mock egg salad.

- Tofu can replace cream or cheese as a base for salad dressing.

Meat, Poultry, and Fish

Tofu

Anything meat, poultry, or fish can do, tofu can also do, but without the cholesterol and a fraction of the fat and calories.

- Tofu can be cubed and added to soups or stews in place of meat, fish, or poultry.

- Frozen tofu that has been defrosted has a meatlike texture. It can be barbecued whole or crumbled into "vegetarian" chili, seasoned with taco seasoning and used as meat substitute in tacos, or cooked into spaghetti sauce in place of ground beef.

- Tofu's light color and texture makes it an excellent chicken substitute in stir-fried dishes, soups, or stews. Tofu works especially well in Italian dishes because it soaks up the spices even better than chicken.

- Tofu can be crumbled into meatloaf to reduce the meat content. (Try mixing 1 pound of tofu to 1 pound extra-lean ground beef.)

- Tofu can be mashed with bread crumbs (or oatmeal), chopped onions, mustard, barbecue sauce, and other seasonings to make a "tofu burger."

- Okara, the by-product of tofu production that is rich in protein and fiber, can be made into a vegetable patty and used in place of meat as a main dish. (Okara patties are sold in many natural food stores. See pages 187–188 for okara recipes.)

Tempeh

Where's the beef? They won't even miss it if you serve tempeh instead—its chewy texture and nutty taste make it a perfect meat substitute.

- Tempeh can be diced and used as a base for mock chicken salad.

- Tempeh can be grilled or cooked as a burger instead of beef.

Textured Soy Protein

Textured soy protein (TSP) can be used in any recipe calling for chopped meat, including hamburgers, meatloaf, tacos, or spaghetti sauce.

- For a more "meaty" flavor, mix equal amounts of rehydrated TSP with lean chopped meat.

- For stews, TSP comes in meat-colored chunks that look (if not taste) like the real thing. For the best results, give the stew plenty of time to simmer so the "meat" picks up the flavor of the vegetables and seasonings.

- Ready-made TSP patties can be purchased in natural food stores and some supermarkets. Put a veggie burger on a bun with ketchup, mustard, pickles, onions, tomato (you can even splurge and use a slice of low-fat cheddar cheese) for a low-fat version of the fast-food favorite.

Meat Analogs

There's a wide variety of mock meat, soybean derived products to suit any palate. Although many of these products are lower in fat, cholesterol, and calories than the real thing, some are laden with additives and preservatives. Read the label carefully!

- Breakfast with soy bacon or meatless sausage.

- Try soy luncheon "meat" or a vegetarian hot dog for lunch. (Put it on a bun with mustard and relish and it takes remarkably similar to a real hot dog.)

- Try a prepared soy entree for dinner, such as "chicken" enchiladas or tofu steak.

Twelve

Cooking With Soy

Here are some tips on storing and cooking soy foods:

Caring for Your Tofu

Fresh tofu is usually stored floating in bins of water at the greengrocer, Asian market, or supermarket. According to tofu expert Dr. Lester Wilson of Iowa State University (who is known as Dr. Tofu among his colleagues), fresh tofu should be refrigerated. Don't buy it unless it is stored in a refrigerated display case! Unrefrigerated fresh tofu can become tainted with the same kinds of microorganisms as attack unrefrigerated meat or milk. Tofu is also pasteurized and sold in packages; although it has a longer shelf life than fresh tofu, pasteurized tofu also needs to be refrigerated. As of this writing, there are two brands of aseptically packaged tofu on the market that do not need to be refrigerated. In terms of taste, if you're eating tofu in its natural form, the fresher the tofu the better. However, after cooking, I find that there is very little difference between fresh or packaged tofu.

Ideally, fresh tofu should be used within five to seven days of when it is made. It can be stored in your refrigerator for up to seven days in water, however be sure to change the water daily. (Some packaged tofu is dated for freshness.)

When cooking with tofu, you may have to use more spices and seasonings than you would cooking with meat. You may have to add as much as double the amount of spices for some recipes.

To freeze tofu, drain it to eliminate excess moisture and wrap it in foil or plastic before placing in the freezer. (To drain tofu, put it between several pieces of paper towel for fifteen minutes; the towels will absorb the excess water.) According to the Soyfoods Association of America, tofu can be frozen for up to five months. Thaw at room temperature. Defrosted tofu will have a slightly brownish color and a chewy texture. Before cooking with defrosted tofu, be sure to squeeze out excess water.

If the tofu develops an unpleasant odor, discard it.

Tempeh

Tempeh should be stored in the freezer or refrigerator; frozen tempeh can keep for several months. If the recipe doesn't require cooking, steam or bake the tempeh for ten minutes before using it in food.

Soy Flour

For freshness, store soy flour in the refrigerator or freezer. Stir the flour before measuring because it can become packed in its container.

Soy flour tends to brown more easily than other flours. Be sure to shorten the baking time or slightly lower the oven temperature of baked goods.

Soy Milk

Soy milk is usually sold in aseptic packages that do not require refrigeration. However, once the package is opened, it should be refrigerated and used within a week.

Texturized Soy Protein

Texturized soy protein must be rehydrated before using. The rehydrated product should be stored in the refrigerator and used within four days.

Thirteen

Breakfast the Soy Way

Eight million Americans start their day with a sugary glass of cola, and half of all Americans don't eat any breakfast at all! Some people complain that they're too rushed to cook in the morning, and some contend that they just can't face solid food right after waking up. If you can't seem to eat breakfast, I've got the perfect solution: try drinking it! A soy shake is a terrific way to begin the day. There are several prepared soy protein powder drinks on the market that come plain or flavored, such as Spiru-tein or Take Care. Simply mix with water or juice and drink. For just a little more effort, you can make your own. Following are five fabulous recipes guaranteed to improve your mornings (when making tofu shakes, add a few drops of lemon juice to eliminate a tofu aftertaste):

Basic High Protein Shake

Serves 1

It doesn't get much easier than this!

1 cup juice of your choice
4 tablespoons soy protein isolate, plain or flavored

Mix in a glass and drink. For a thicker, creamier beverage, process ingredients in a blender until smooth. For extra froth, add 2 or 3 ice cubes before blending.

High Protein "Milk" Shake

Serves 1

1 cup soy milk (Westbrae 1% Lite vanilla is particularly good)
½ teaspoon carob powder
Pinch of ground cinnamon
Crushed ice

Process ingredients in a blender until smooth. Pour into a glass and drink.

Basic Fruit Smoothie

Serves 3

1 package 10½ ounces soft low-fat tofu
1 cup 100 percent fruit juice
1 teaspoon lemon juice
1 cup chopped fresh fruit
2 tablespoons honey or to taste
8 ice cubes

Place the tofu, juices, fruit, honey, and ice cubes in a blender.
Process until smooth. Pour into glasses and serve.

SOURCE: Judith Eaton and Karen Lefkowitz

Tofu Fruit Shake

Serves 1

1/4 cup soft tofu
1/2 cup fruit juice
1/2 banana
1/2 tablespoon honey
1/2 teaspoon vanilla extract
1/4 cup partially thawed chopped frozen fruit

Mix ingredients in a blender, processing until smooth. Pour
into a glass and drink.

SOURCE: Adapted from a recipe by Bountiful Bean Soyfoods

Creamy Banana Date Shake

Serves 1

1/2 cup apple juice
1/4 cup soft tofu
2 pitted dates
1/2 banana

Mix ingredients in a blender, processing until smooth. Serve chilled.

SOURCE: Soyfoods Association of America, with funding from the United Soybean Board

Raspberry Kiwi Delight

Serves 1

1/4 cup soft tofu
1/4 cup frozen raspberries
1/2 kiwi
1/2 cup orange or pineapple juice

Mix the ingredients in a blender, processing until smooth. Pour into a glass and drink.

Part V

SEVENTY SUPER SOY RECIPES

Introduction

Want to know how to get more soy into your life? This part of the book contains seventy recipes for appetizers, soups, main courses, and desserts—all based on soy products and all good tasting. Many of these recipes were developed by nutritionists Judith Eaton, M.S., R.D., and Karen Lefkowitz, M.S., who, as they say, have been carrying the tofu torch for many years. Judith and Karen run Nutrition Services, a consulting firm in Pomona, New York, with clients ranging from industry to private patients. Judith is the prenatal nutrition consultant for Phelps Memorial Hospital in New York and for Planned Parenthood, and a nutrition consultant for the American Health Foundation. Karen is a nutrition consultant for the Child Health Center of the American Health Foundation. She has also served as a consultant for the Pediatric Department of New York Medical College. Judith and Karen have devoted a great deal of their professional time to solving the nutritional problems of children and teenagers. They are coordinators of the American Health Foundation's Bodybeat Program, a weight-management program for young adolescents and have worked with children with high cholesterol.

In order to reduce fat, Judith and Karen use Mori-Nu brand's low-fat tofu in their recipes. If you substitute other tofus, remember it will add a few more fat grams and calories. (A 4-ounce serving of regular firm tofu contains 6 grams of fat and 120 calories; regular soft tofu contains 5 fat grams and 86 calories; regular silken tofu contains 2.4 fat grams and 72 calories.)

I have also collected terrific recipes from other sources. Macrobiotic cook Ana McIntyre, a well-known spa chef, contributed three of her unique soy recipes.

Lynne Paterson, product development consultant to Lightlife Foods, is an internationally recognized cooking teacher, caterer, and frequent contributor to *Natural Health Magazine*. Ms. Paterson, a professional chef and owner of Valley Natural Foodservices of Shutesbury, Massachusetts, contributed an original soyfood recipe to this book. In addition, some soy food producers were kind enough to share their best recipes.

Several producers of high-quality soyfood products, including Vitasoy, Eden Foods, Azumaya, Bountiful Bean Soyfoods, and Worthington Foods (marketed under the brand name Natural Touch) also contributed some excellent recipes. Their products can be found at natural food stores and many supermarkets In addition, we received some terrific recipes from the Soyfoods Association of America, the United Soybean Board, the Missouri Soybean Board, and Soy Ohio. Many of these soyfood manufacturers and trade associations will provide additional recipes free of charge. (For more information, see Resources, page 234.)

In some recipes, we specify that a low-fat or no-fat version of a particular ingredient, or a no-salt or salt-reduced ingredient, is preferred. Keep in mind that the nutritional analysis is based on the lowest fat, lowest salt product. In addition, we did not include optional ingredients, or optional accompaniment such as bread, crackers, or chips, in the analysis. Unless otherwise specified, use medium-size fruits and vegetables in the recipes.

The following recipes are included:

Salads

Curried Tofu Rice Salad
Vegetable Couscous with Tofu
Tofu Mock Egg Salad
Tempeh Mock Chicken Salad

Spreads, Dressings, and Sauces

Peanut Butter and Jelly Lover's Tofu Spread
Tofu Tuna Spread
Savory Cheese Spread
Herbed Tofu Pâté
Tofu Ginger-Peanut Dressing
Sweet Poppy Dressing
Tofu Mole Dip
Zesty Cilantro Dip
Creamy White Sauce
Cholesterol-Free Hollandaise Sauce

Soups

Cream of Cauliflower Soup
Spicy Carrot Soup

Crabmeat and Asparagus Soup
Tofu and Corn Bisque
Cream of Vegetable Soup
Miso Soup with Onions

Main Dishes

Tofu Sloppy Joes
Sloppy Joes with Texturized Soy Protein
Fusilli and Tofu with Sauce Verde
Tofu Meatballs
Tofu Cutlets Parmesan
Tofu Stuffed Pepper
Quinoa with Tofu
Crustless Onion-Mushroom Quiche
Athenian Tofu
Okara Patties with Spicy Peanut Sauce
Okara Patty Foo Yong
Tempeh Pizza
Busy Day Chili
Sweet-and-Sour Hawaiian Tempeh
Quick-and-Easy Spinach Lasagna
Tempeh Reuben Sandwiches
Barbecued Tofu
Tofu with Condiments
Sesame Tofu
Noodle Pudding
Tempeh-Lemon Broil
Barbecued Grilled Tempeh with Onions
Tex-Mex Tempeh

Rice and Tofu Loaf
Tofu and Mushrooms
Tofu Rice Stir-Fry
Tofu Bouillabaisse
Chicken Tetrazzini
Chicken and Tofu Stir-Fry
Chicken Paprika
Beefy Tofu Enchiladas
Meat Loaf

Breads and Breakfasts

Peach Breakfast Soufflé
Toffins
Zucchini Bread
Eastern Omelet
Apple Pancakes
Banana Pancakes

Desserts

Chocolate Tofu Berry Whip
Chocolate Chip Cookies
Chocolate Cream Pie
Tofu Brownies
Tofu Strawberry Cheese Cake
Creamsicle Spritzer
Tofu Pumpkin Pie
Strawberry Fluff
Super-Moist Carrot Cake

Vanilla Pudding
Piña Colada
Low Cal Chocolate Mousse

Salads

Curried Tofu Rice Salad

Serves 4

1 package (10½ ounces) firm or extra-firm low-fat tofu,
    drained
1½ cups cooked brown rice
2 scallions, finely chopped
1 tablespoon finely chopped fresh parsley
1 tomato, diced

DRESSING

½ tablespoon lemon juice
½ teaspoon curry powder
⅛ teaspoon chili powder
½ teaspoon garlic powder
¼ teaspoon salt
⅛ teaspoon ground black pepper
1 tablespoon olive oil
2½ tablespoons vinegar

GARNISH

Lettuce leaves
Sliced cucumbers
Sliced red and green bell peppers

1. Slice the tofu and drain between several layers of paper towels for 15 to 20 minutes. Remove tofu and crumble into small pieces and place in bowl. Add the rice, scallions, parsley, and tomato and mix well.

2. Mix seasonings for dressing with oil. Toss with tofu-rice mixture, then toss with vinegar. Let marinate from 30 minutes to several hours in the refrigerator.

3. Serve on lettuce leaves and garnish with slices of cucumbers and red and green peppers.

PER SERVING Calories: 154   Fat: 5 g
         Saturated fat: under 1 g   Fiber: 2 g
         Cholesterol: 0   Sodium: 209 mg
         Calcium: 29 mg   Iron: 6 mg

RESOURCE: Judith Eaton and Karen Lefkowitz

Vegetable Couscous with Tofu

Serves 6

2 packages (10½ ounces each) extra-firm low-fat tofu
1 large onion, chopped
1 large red bell pepper, chopped
4 carrots, thinly sliced
2 zucchini, sliced in ½-inch pieces
1 can (15 ounces) navy beans, rinsed and drained
1½ cups tomato sauce, preferably low salt
1½ cups low-salt, fat-free chicken broth
½ cup raisins
2 teaspoons curry powder
¼ teaspoon cayenne pepper
1 teaspoon paprika
1¾ cups couscous

1. Cut the tofu into ½-inch cubes. Drain in colander.

2. Spray a heavy, large skillet with nonstick cooking spray. Add the onion, pepper, carrots, and tofu. Sauté for 10 minutes, stirring occasionally.

3. Add the zucchini and cook an additional 2 minutes.

4. Add the beans, tomato sauce, broth, raisins, curry powder, cayenne, and paprika. Cover and bring to boil. Simmer for 30 minutes.

5. Prepare couscous according to package directions. Serve cooked vegetables over couscous.

PER SERVING Calories: 433   Fat: 2.5 g
             Saturated fat: under 2 g   Fiber: 12 g
             Cholesterol: 0   Sodium: 538 mg
             Calcium: 108 mg   Iron: 10.6 mg
RESOURCE: Judith Eaton and Karen Lefkowitz

Tofu Mock Egg Salad

Serves 4

1 pound firm tofu
1 tablespoon low-sodium soy sauce
¾ teaspoon prepared mustard
¼ teaspoon garlic powder
¼ teaspoon curry powder
Pinch of cayenne pepper
1 tablespoon minced fresh parsley
1 small celery stalk, chopped
1 tablespoon minced onion
2 tablespoons mayonnaise, preferably reduced-fat
2 tablespoons honey
1 tablespoon lemon juice

1. Mash the tofu with a fork in a large bowl.

2. Combine with remaining ingredients and mix well. Adjust seasonings to taste.

3. Spread on bread, toast or crackers, or serve as a vegetable dip.

PER SERVING	Calories: 176	Fat: 7 g
(NOT INCLUD-	Saturated fat: 1 g	Fiber: less than 1 g
ING ACCOMPA-	Cholesterol: 2.5 mg	Sodium: 171 mg
NIMENTS)	Calcium: 128 mg	Iron: 6.4 mg

RESOURCE: Bountiful Bean Soyfoods

Tempeh Mock Chicken Salad

Serves 2

1 cup water
8 ounces tempeh, cut in 1-inch pieces
1 bay leaf
1 tablespoon sesame tahini
1 tablespoon white miso
1 teaspoon prepared mustard
1 celery stalk, finely diced
¼ cup minced scallions

1. In a small saucepan, bring water to a boil. Add the tempeh and bay leaf. Cover, reduce heat, and simmer for about 20 minutes.

2. Remove the lid and boil off remaining water. Let tempeh cool.

3. In a bowl, mash the tempeh with the tahini, miso, and mustard. Mix in the celery and scallions. Refrigerate for several hours.

4. Serve as a side-dish salad on lettuce leaves or as a filling for sandwiches or pita pockets.

PER SERVING   Calories: 270   Fat: 15 g
                Saturated fat: less than 1 g   Fiber: 5 g
                Cholesterol: 0   Sodium: 377 mg
                Calcium: 122 mg   Iron: 3 mg
RESOURCE: Ana McIntyre

Spreads, Dressings, and Sauces

Peanut Butter and Jelly Lover's Tofu Spread

Serves 3

Love PB and J but hate the fat? Try this lower-fat version on bread or crackers.

1 package (10½ ounces) firm low-fat tofu
3 tablespoons natural-style chunky peanut butter
¼ cup black raspberry all-fruit preserves

1. Drain the tofu.

2. Place the tofu and peanut butter in a food processor and process until smooth.

3. Add the preserves and process with on/off motion until blended. Chill for several hours to allow flavors to blend.

PER SERVING Calories: 180   Fat: 8 g
             Saturated fat: 1 g   Fiber: 1 g
             Cholesterol: 0   Sodium: 95 mg
             Calcium: 23 mg   Iron: 7 mg
RESOURCE: Judith Eaton and Karen Lefkowitz

Tofu Tuna Spread

Serve as a sandwich spread or with crackers and crudités.

Serves 4

1 package (10½ ounces) firm or extra-firm low-fat tofu
1 can (6⅛ ounces) tuna, packed in water
1 small purple onion
½ cup grated carrot
¼ cup chopped fresh parsley
1 tablespoon fat-free mayonnaise or soy mayonnaise
2 tablespoons honey mustard

1. Drain the tofu and tuna.

2. In a food processor, chop the onion.

3. Add the tofu and tuna and process until desired consistency. Stir in the carrots and parsley.

4. In a small bowl, mix the mayonnaise and mustard, then blend into the tuna mixture.

PER SERVING   Calories: 84   Fat: 2.5 g
                       Saturated fat: less than 1 g   Fiber: 1 g
                       Cholesterol: 5 g   Sodium: 106 mg
                       Calcium: 28 mg   Iron: 1 mg
RESOURCE: Judith Eaton and Karen Lefkowitz

Savory Cheese Spread

Makes 36 1-tablespoon servings

½ cup grated reduced-fat, low-salt cheddar cheese
½ cup grated Parmesan cheese
½ cup mashed tofu
½ cup mayonnaise, preferably reduced-fat
¼ cup diced pitted green olives
2 tablespoons grated onion
2 tablespoons chopped fresh parsley
1 teaspoon curry powder
Party rye slices

1. Combine all the ingredients in mixing bowl.

2. Spread on party rye and serve.

PER SERVING   Calories: 24   Fat: 2 g
                       Saturated fat: under 1 g   Fiber: 0
                       Cholesterol: 3 mg   Sodium: 58 mg
                       Calcium: 35 mg   Iron: less than 1 mg
RESOURCE: Missouri Soybean Board

Herbed Tofu Pâté

Makes 36 1-tablespoon servings

1 pound firm tofu, drained
1 tablespoon white miso
1 tablespoon sesame tahini
1 teaspoon umeboshi plum paste
1 teaspoon fresh lemon juice
1 tablespoon minced chives
1 tablespoon minced fresh basil

1. Drain excess water from the tofu by either slicing and pressing under a weight or wringing out in a clean cotton towel.

2. Place all ingredients in a mixing bowl and mash thoroughly until smooth.

3. Press the mixture into a mold and refrigerate for several hours or overnight to let the flavors blend.

4. Slice or scoop out and serve on sandwiches or crackers for a tasty, lower-fat alternative to a cream cheese spread.

PER SERVING Calories: 14   Fat: 1 g
             Saturated fat: less than 1 g   Fiber: less than 1 g
             Cholesterol: 0   Sodium: 18 mg
             Calcium: 14 mg   Iron: less than 1 mg
RESOURCE· Ana McIntyre

Tofu Ginger-Peanut Dressing

This sauce is terrific on oriental chicken salad, raw veggies, steamed vegetables, or salad greens. Mix with whole wheat or buckwheat noodles for a lunch kids really enjoy. It will stay fresh in the refrigerator for up to one week.

Serves 12

3 scallions (white part only)
3-inch piece fresh ginger, peeled
2 garlic cloves
3 tablespoons natural-style peanut butter, smooth or chunky
2 packages (10½ ounces) firm low-fat tofu
1 teaspoon dark roasted sesame oil
⅓ cup low-sodium soy sauce
¼ cup honey
1 cup rice wine vinegar
2 cups water

1. Process the scallions, ginger, and garlic in a food processor or blender until smooth.

2. Add the peanut butter, tofu, sesame oil, soy sauce, and honey; process until the mixture is blended.

3. Slowly add the vinegar and water, and process until blended.

PER SERVING Calories: 75   Fat: 2.5 g
           Saturated fat: under 1 g   Fiber: under 1 g
           Cholesterol: 12 mg   Sodium: 299 mg
           Calcium: 16 mg   Iron: 4 mg
RESOURCE: Judith Eaton and Karen Lefkowitz

Sweet Poppy Dressing

Serves 8

2 tablespoons Dijon-style mustard
2 tablespoons honey
Juice of 1 lemon
1 cup Light Original Vitasoy
2 teaspoons poppy seeds
½ teaspoon paprika
¼ teaspoon grated orange zest

1. Mix the mustard and honey in a bowl.

2. Slowly blend in the lemon juice and soy milk. Add the remaining ingredients.

3. Use to dress a crisp green salad or as a vegetable dip.

PER SERVING Calories: 72   Fat: 3g
             Saturated fat: less than 1g   Fiber: 0
             Cholesterol: 0   Sodium: 629 mg
             Calcium: 46 mg   Iron: 0
RESOURCE: Vitasoy, Inc.

Tofu Mole Dip

Makes 37 1-tablespoon servings

1 package (10½ ounces) soft tofu, drained
1½ teaspoons lemon juice
1 teaspoon garlic powder
2 tablespoons diced onion
2 tablespoons chopped fresh cilantro
½ teaspoon chili powder
1 small tomato, diced
1 ripe medium avocado, mashed

1. In a blender or food processor, combine the tofu, lemon juice, garlic powder, onion, cilantro, and chili powder until well blended.

2. Put the mixture in a serving bowl. Add the tomato and avocado, and mix well. Chill and serve with no-fat chips or fresh vegetables.

PER SERVING Calories: 19   Fat: 1 g
             Saturated fat: less than 1 g   Fiber: less than 1 g
             Cholesterol: 0   Sodium: 3 mg
             Calcium: 4.7 mg   Iron: less than 1 mg
RESOURCE: Missouri Soybean Board

Zesty Cilantro Dip

Serves 8

½ cup chopped fresh cilantro
1 can (4 ounces) green chilies, diced and drained
2 cups frozen petite peas, thawed
1 package (10½ ounces) low-fat firm tofu, drained
1 tablespoon lemon juice
1½ teaspoons ground cumin
¼ teaspoon freshly ground pepper
Salt to taste (optional)

2 tomatoes, sliced
4 cups sliced raw vegetables of choice

1. In a food processor or blender, combine ¼ cup cilantro and all the dip ingredients until smooth, blending approximately 30 seconds on high. Refrigerate for 1 hour.

2. Mound on overlapping tomato slices and rim with fresh cilantro. Serve with vegetables.

PER SERVING Calories: 62 g   Fat: 1 g
             Saturated fat: less than 1 g   Fiber: 0
             Cholesterol: 0   Sodium: 50 mg
             Calcium: 30 mg   Iron: 1 mg
RESOURCE: Mori-nu

Creamy White Sauce

Serves 4

1 tablespoon vegetable oil
1½ tablespoons organic unbleached white flour
1½ cups Edensoy Original Organic soy milk
½ teaspoon sea salt
2 large garlic cloves, crushed
2 teaspoons mirin (rice wine)
2 tablespoons finely chopped fresh parsley

1. Mix the oil and flour in a heavy saucepan. Warm over low heat, stirring constantly, for 3 to 5 minutes. Slowly add the soy milk, stirring constantly as sauce thickens.

2. Add salt, garlic, and mirin. Simmer uncovered over low heat, stirring occasionally for 10 to 15 minutes. Remove from heat and stir in parsley.

3. Serve over pasta.

PER SERVING Calories: 75   Fat: 9 g
            Saturated fat: less than 1 g   Fiber: less than 1 g
            Cholesterol: 0   Sodium: 280 mg
            Calcium: 11 mg   Iron: less than 1 mg
RESOURCE: Eden Foods

Cholesterol-Free Hollandaise Sauce

This eggless hollandaise is delicious over cooked vegetables, fish, tempeh, tofu, or seafood.

Serves 4

1 cup Edensoy Original Organic soy milk
2 tablespoons corn oil
¼ teaspoon sea salt
1 tablespoon kudzu or cornstarch, dissolved in 2 tablespoons water
1 tablespoon lemon juice
Paprika or ground nutmeg, for garnish

1. Combine the soy milk, oil, salt, and kudzu or cornstarch mixture in a saucepan. Simmer for 3 to 5 minutes, stirring constantly with wire whisk, until mixture becomes thick.

2. Add lemon juice to sauce, then pour over hot food. Garnish with paprika or nutmeg.

PER SERVING Calories: 90   Fat: 8 g
             Saturated fat: less than 1 g   Fiber: 0
             Cholesterol: 0   Sodium: 140 mg
             Calcium: 4 mg   Iron: less than 1 mg
RESOURCE: Eden Foods

Soups

Cream of Cauliflower Soup

Serves 8

1 large cauliflower
2 teaspoons canola oil
1 onion, chopped
3 celery stalks, chopped
¼ cup all-purpose flour
4 cups fat-free, low-salt chicken broth, canned or homemade
1 package (10½ ounces) soft low-fat tofu
1 cup skim milk
1 teaspoon paprika
1 teaspoon grated nutmeg
Salt and pepper to taste (optional)
Grated Parmesan cheese, preferably fat-free cheese alternative (optional)

1. Cut the cauliflower into florets and remove stems. Steam lightly for 12 minutes or microwave on high for 5 to 7 minutes.

2. Drain the cauliflower and reserve about one third of the florets. Puree the remaining florets in a blender or food processor.

3. In a large pot, heat the oil and sauté the onion and celery until tender, about 5 minutes.

4. Add the flour to the vegetables and stir. Slowly add the chicken broth and bring to a boil. Mix in the pureed cauliflower and reduce heat to a simmer.

5. In a blender or food processor, blend the tofu and milk. Slowly add this mixture to soup.

6. Add the reserved florets, paprika, nutmeg, and optional salt and pepper. Pour into serving bowls and, if desired, add a sprinkling of Parmesan cheese.

PER SERVING Calories: 97   Fat: 3 g
             Saturated fat: under 1 g   Fiber: 3 g
             Cholesterol: under 1 mg   Sodium: 235 mg
             Calcium: 83 mg   Iron: 1 mg
RESOURCE: Judith Eaton and Karen Lefkowitz

Spicy Carrot Soup

Serves 4

1 tablespoon olive oil
1 small onion, chopped
4 large carrots, chopped
1 garlic clove, minced
¼ teaspoon mustard seeds
¼ teaspoon ground ginger
¼ teaspoon ground cumin
¼ teaspoon turmeric
Pinch of ground cinnamon
Pinch of cayenne pepper
¼ teaspoon salt
½ tablespoon lemon juice

½ cup water

2 tablespoons unsalted margarine

2 tablespoons whole wheat flour

2 packages (16.8 ounces each) Creamy Original Vitasoy soy
  milk

½ teaspoon honey

¼ cup low-fat yogurt

1. In a large saucepan, heat the olive oil and sauté the onion until golden, about 3 minutes. Add the carrots, garlic, mustard seeds, spices, salt, and lemon juice. Cook for 2 to 3 minutes, stirring constantly.

2. Add the water, cover, and simmer for 20 minutes or until carrots are tender. Let cool.

3. Place the mixture in a blender and puree on low speed until smooth.

4. In a sauce pan, melt the margarine, add the flour, and cook for 2 to 3 minutes, stirring constantly. Whisk in the soy milk, then add the carrot puree and cook for 10 minutes, stirring constantly. Serve hot with a spoonful of yogurt on top.

PER SERVING Calories: 182   Fat: 10 g

             Saturated fat: 2 g   Fiber: 3 g

             Cholesterol: 0   Sodium: 159 mg

             Calcium: 75 mg   Iron: less than 1 mg

RESOURCE: Vitasoy, Inc.

Crabmeat and Asparagus Soup

Serves 3

½ pound fresh asparagus
1 tablespoon unsalted margarine
¼ cup finely chopped onion
2 tablespoons whole wheat flour
2 packages (16.8 ounces) Creamy Original Vitasoy soy milk
¼ teaspoon salt
pinch each of black pepper, paprika, garlic powder, and
    ground nutmeg
½ pound fresh asparagus
¼ pound lump crabmeat

1. Wash the asparagus well. Steam until tender, about 15 minutes, then chop and drain.

2. In a large saucepan, melt the margarine over medium heat. Stir in onion and sauté until golden, about 3 minutes. Add the flour and cook the mixture for 2 to 3 minutes, stirring constantly.

3. Gradually whisk in the soy milk, then add the salt and other seasonings, stirring constantly.

4. Add the asparagus, reduce heat to low, and cook for 5 minutes.

5. Add the crabmeat and bring the soup to boil. Serve immediately.

PER SERVING Calories: 175   Fat: 7 g
             Saturated fat: 1 g   Fiber: 2 g
             Cholesterol: 39 mg   Sodium: 370 mg
             Calcium: 84 mg   Iron: 1 mg
RESOURCE: Vitasoy, Inc.

Tofu and Corn Bisque

Serves 8

4 tablespoons unsalted margarine
2 small onions, finely chopped
2 teaspoons mild curry powder
2 teaspoons paprika
½ cup all-purpose flour
4 cups vegetable stock
1 package (33.8 ounces) Light Original Vitasoy soy milk
Grated rind of 1 lemon
1 large can (24 ounces) whole kernel corn, drained
1 package (16 ounces) firm tofu, drained and cubed
2 tablespoons chopped fresh parsley

1. Melt margarine in a large saucepan and gently cook the onions until soft, about 5 minutes.

2. Stir in the curry powder, paprika, and flour and cook for 1 minute. Gradually add the stock and bring to boil, stirring constantly.

3. Stir in the soy milk, lemon rind, and corn. Simmer for 5 minutes.

4. Stir in tofu and simmer for 5 minutes. Garnish with parsley.

PER SERVING Calories: 386   Fat: 17 g
                        Saturated fat: 3 g   Fiber: 3 g
                        Cholesterol: 4 mg   Sodium: 626 mg
                        Calcium: 191 mg   Iron: 8 mg
RESOURCE: Vitasoy, Inc.

Cream of Vegetable Soup

Any leftover vegetables can be used in this soup!

Serves 10

2 teaspoons olive oil

1 cup chopped onion

2 garlic cloves, minced

4 carrots, chopped

2 celery stalks, chopped

2 cups shredded green cabbage

1 can (2 pounds, 3 ounces) Italian-style plum tomatoes

4 cups fat-free, low-salt canned chicken broth, or 4 cups
     homemade chicken stock

2 tablespoons chopped fresh parsley, or 2 teaspoons dried

2 tablespoons chopped fresh dill, or 2 teaspoons dried

2 tablespoons chopped fresh basil, or 2 teaspoons dried

1 teaspoon dried oregano

1 tablespoon sugar

Salt and pepper to taste (optional)

1 package (10½ ounces) soft low-fat tofu

1. In a large, heavy pot, heat the olive oil over medium heat. Add the onions and garlic and cook for 3 minutes.

2. Add the carrots, celery, and cabbage and sauté briefly, 2 to 3 minutes.

3. Add the tomatoes and chicken broth. Stir in the parsley, dill, basil, oregano, sugar, and optional salt and pepper. Bring to boil, lower heat and simmer for 1 hour.

4. Carefully, 1 cup at a time, puree the soup in a blender or food processor. Return soup to pot.

5. Blend the tofu in a blender or food processor. Slowly add tofu to soup and mix well. Heat soup thoroughly.

PER SERVING	Calories: 84	Fat: 2.6 g
	Saturated fat: under 1 g	Fiber: 2.5 g
	Cholesterol: 0	Sodium: 322 mg
	Calcium: 64 mg	Iron: 1.5 mg

RESOURCE: Judith Eaton and Karen Lefkowitz

Miso Soup with Onions

Serves 4

4 cups water

1 cup sliced onion

1 low-sodium bouillon cube (chicken, vegetable, or beef)

1 package (10½ ounces) extra-firm low-fat tofu, diced

½ tablespoon low-sodium soy sauce

1 tablespoon dark miso, diluted in a little soup stock

½ cup nori (dried seaweed)

2 scallions, thinly sliced

1. Place the water in a large pot and bring to boil over medium heat. Add the onion and bouillon cube; simmer for 2 minutes.

2. Add the tofu and soy sauce; simmer 5 minutes.

3. Add the diluted miso and stir gently. Turn heat to low and simmer for 2 to 3 minutes.

4. Lightly toast the *nori* over an open flame or stove burner until the color changes; crumble and add to soup.

5. Serve and garnish with scallions.

PER SERVING		
	Calories: 65	Fat: 1 g
	Saturated fat: under 1 g	Fiber: 1.3 g
	Cholesterol: 0	Sodium: 399 mg
	Calcium: 43 mg	Iron: 6 mg

RESOURCE: Judith Eaton and Karen Lefkowitz

Main Dishes

Tofu Sloppy Joes

Serves 3

3 English muffins, preferably whole grain, split in halves
1 package (10½ ounces) soft or firm low-fat tofu, drained
½ cup fat-free, salt-reduced, meatless spaghetti sauce
1½ teaspoons grated Parmesan cheese
6 tablespoons shredded reduced-fat mozzarella, or reduced-fat soy cheese

1. Toast the muffins until lightly browned.

2. Place the tofu in a nonstick frying pan and mash with a potato masher or fork. Cook over high heat for 5 minutes, stirring occasionally.

3. Add the pasta sauce and continue cooking over high heat for 4 minutes, stirring occasionally.

4. Divide the tofu mixture among the 6 muffin halves and sprinkle each with ¼ teaspoon Parmesan cheese.

5. Top each with a tablespoon of mozzarella cheese.

6. Place on a microwave-safe plate and cook on high in microwave for 2½ minutes or until cheese has melted.

PER SERVING Calories: 240   Fat: 7 g

Saturated fat: under 1 g   Fiber: 2 g

Cholesterol: 9 mg   Sodium: 477 mg

Calcium: 106 mg   Iron: 3.3 mg

RESOURCE: Judith Eaton and Karen Lefkowitz

Sloppy Joes with Texturized Soy Protein

Serves 4

⅞ cup boiling water
1 cup dry texturized soy protein
1 cup chopped onion
1 large green bell pepper, coarsely chopped
3 tablespoons soybean or canola oil
2 cups low-salt tomato sauce
1–1½ tablespoons chili powder
1 tablespoon low-sodium soy sauce
2 tablespoons sugar
Salt and pepper to taste
4 hamburger rolls, split in halves

1. Pour boiling water over the texturized soy protein and set aside.

2. In a large pan, sauté the onion and green pepper in the oil until they are tender, about 5 minutes.

3. Add the texturized soy protein and the rest of the ingredients. Simmer for 20 minutes.

4. Serve over split hamburger rolls.

PER SERVING Calories: 371   Fat: 13 g
             Saturated fat: 2 g   Fiber: 8 g
             Cholesterol: 0   Sodium: 457 mg
             Calcium: 169 mg   Iron: 5 mg
RESOURCE: Adapted from a recipe developed by the United Soybean Board

Fusilli and Tofu with Sauce Verde

Serves 4

1 package (8 ounces) fusilli (corkscrew) pasta
1 package (10½ ounces) extra-firm low-fat tofu, drained and
    cut in ½-inch cubes
1–2 garlic cloves
½ cup chopped fresh parsley
½ cup chopped fresh cilantro
3 scallions
¼ cup grated Parmesan cheese, preferably fat-free cheese
    alternative
1 tablespoon olive oil
2 teaspoons sesame tahini
1 cup chopped raw broccoli

1. Prepare the pasta according to directions on the package.
Drain and place in a medium bowl. Add the tofu.

2. Place the garlic, parsley, cilantro, scallions, cheese, olive oil
and tahini in a food processor. Process until smooth. Add to
the pasta and tofu.

3. Process the broccoli with an on/off motion until it is coarsely
chopped. Add to pasta mixture. Toss well. Serve warm or cold.

PER SERVING Calories: 329   Fat: 8 g
             Saturated fat: less than 1 g   Fiber: 1 g
             Cholesterol: 0   Sodium: 150 mg
             Calcium: 64 mg   Iron: 9 mg
RESOURCE: Judith Eaton and Karen Lefkowitz

Tofu Meatballs

Serves 4

1 large onion

1 cup chopped fresh curly parsley

2 packages (10½ ounces each) extra-firm low-fat tofu, drained

½ cup seasoned bread crumbs

½ cup egg substitute

½ teaspoon dried basil

½ teaspoon dried minced garlic

½ teaspoon dried oregano

½ teaspoon black pepper

½ teaspoon dry mustard

¼ teaspoon fennel seeds

¼ teaspoon ground nutmeg

¼ cup grated Parmesan cheese, preferably fat-free cheese alternative

1½ cups plus 3 tablespoons tomato sauce, preferably low-salt

¼ cup whole wheat flour

1. Preheat the oven to 350° F.

2. Place the onion and parsley in a food processor. Process until smooth.

3. Add the tofu, bread crumbs, egg substitute, herbs, pepper, mustard, fennel, nutmeg, cheese, and 3 tablespoons of tomato sauce. Process with on/off motion until ingredients are combined.

4. Form 16 balls the size of a walnut, then dust each with flour.

5. Coat nonstick baking pan with nonstick cooking spray. Place the balls in the pan and bake for 35 minutes.

6. Transfer balls to a large nonstick skillet that has been sprayed with nonstick cooking spray. Add the remaining tomato sauce, cover, and simmer 10 to 15 minutes or until sauce is hot.

PER SERVING   Calories: 237   Fat: 4 g
              Saturated fat: under 1 g   Fiber: 3 g
              Cholesterol: 0   Sodium: 436 mg
              Calcium: 140 mg   Iron: 5 mg
RESOURCE: Judith Eaton and Karen Lefkowitz

Tofu Cutlets Parmesan

Serves 6

1 onion, chopped

2 cups tomato sauce, preferably low-salt

1 teaspoon garlic powder

1 teaspoon dried oregano

2 packages (10½ ounces each) extra-firm low-fat tofu

½ cup egg substitute

¾ cup Italian-seasoned bread crumbs

4 ounces reduced-fat mozzarella cheese, grated

4 ounces Parmesan cheese, preferably fat-free cheese alternative, grated

1. Preheat the oven to 350° F.

2. Coat a large skillet with nonstick cooking spray, then sauté onion until wilted, about 3 minutes.

3. Put tomato sauce in a saucepan and add the onion and seasonings. Simmer for 15 minutes.

4. Meanwhile, slice each cake of tofu lengthwise into 3 pieces. Drain on paper towels for 15 minutes.

5. Heat a medium skillet. Dip each tofu slice in egg substitute, then coat with bread crumbs. Fry until delicately brown, about 3 to 4 minutes.

6. Line a baking pan with a little sauce and then layer in the cutlets, adding more sauce and some grated cheese between the layers, leaving some cheese for sprinkling on top. Bake for 20 minutes or until heated through and the cheese has melted.

PER SERVING Calories: 188   Fat: 4 g
             Saturated fat: under 1 g   Fiber: 1.5 g
             Cholesterol: 7 mg   Sodium: 652 mg
             Calcium: 60 mg   Iron: 9 mg
RESOURCE: Judith Eaton and Karen Lefkowitz

Tofu Stuffed Pepper

Serves 5

1 cup cooked brown rice

5 green bell peppers

1 package (10½ ounces) extra-firm low-fat tofu, drained and diced

¼ cup low-sodium soy sauce

1 teaspoon garlic powder

2 small onions

1 celery stalk

2 tablespoons sesame tahini

1 jar (2 ounces) pimiento, drained and chopped
1 cup warm water
1 low-sodium bouillon cube

1. Cook the rice according to package directions.

2. Preheat the oven to 350° F.

3. Remove the seeds and membranes from the peppers, then cut each in half lengthwise.

4. Parboil the peppers for 10 minutes or until nearly tender.

5. While peppers are cooking, marinate the tofu in the soy sauce and garlic powder for 10 minutes.

6. Chop the onions and celery, then spray a skillet with non-stick cooking spray and sauté until tender, about 5 minutes.

7. Mix the rice, celery, and onion with the tahini and pimiento. Stuff the pepper halves with this mixture and then place peppers in roasting pan.

8. Dissolve the bouillon cube in the warm water and pour in roasting pan around the peppers. Bake for 10 to 15 minutes, or until peppers are soft and stuffing is hot.

PER SERVING Calories: 328   Fat: 4 g
　　　　　　Saturated fat: under 1 g   Fiber: 8 g
　　　　　　Cholesterol: under 1 g   Sodium: 362 mg
　　　　　　Calcium: 91 mg   Iron: 75 mg
RESOURCE: Judith Eaton and Karen Lefkowitz

Quinoa with Tofu

Serves 5

1 package (10½ ounces) extra-firm low-fat tofu
½ cup low-sodium teriyaki sauce
1 cup quinoa
2 cups water
2 teaspoons canola oil
1 teaspoon minced fresh ginger
1 onion, minced
3 celery stalks, chopped
2 tablespoons low-sodium soy sauce
1 cup frozen mixed vegetables, thawed

1. Cut the tofu into small cubes and marinate in teriyaki sauce for at least 30 minutes.

2. Rinse the quinoa several times by running fresh water over it in a pot and pouring through a strainer.

3. In a saucepan, bring 2 cups of water to a boil. Add the quinoa, reduce the heat, cover, and simmer until all water is absorbed, 15 to 20 minutes. Set aside.

4. Heat the oil in a large nonstick skillet. Add the ginger and stir. Add the onion and celery, and cook until lightly browned, about 5 minutes.

5. Add the cooked quinoa, soy sauce, and marinated tofu to the skillet. Stir once, cover, and cook for 5 minutes.

6. Add the vegetables. Cook for 2 minutes, covered, or until vegetables are heated through. Do not overcook.

PER SERVING Calories: 215   Fat: 5 g
            Saturated fat: under 1 g   Fiber: 3 g
            Cholesterol: 0   Sodium: 470 mg
            Calcium: 53 mg   Iron: 8 mg
RESOURCE: Judith Eaton and Karen Lefkowitz

Crustless Onion-Mushroom Quiche

Serves 4

1 teaspoon canola oil

2 cups minced onions

2 cups minced fresh mushrooms, plus sliced mushrooms for garnish

¼ teaspoon salt

1½ cups egg substitute

½ cup skim milk or low-fat soy milk

1 package (10½ ounces) firm low-fat tofu

3 ounces grated reduced-fat Jarlsberg or Swiss cheese

1. Preheat the oven to 350° F.

2. In a large nonstick frying pan, heat the oil and cook the onions until lightly browned, about 5 minutes.

3. Add the minced mushrooms and cook over high heat for about 3 minutes. Sprinkle with salt and cook until the mushroom mixture is almost dry. Remove from pan and set aside.

4. In a food processor, blend the egg substitute, milk, and tofu. Add the cheese and mushroom mixture and stir well.

5. Spray a 10-inch quiche dish or pie pan with nonstick spray. Pour the mixture into the prepared pan and decorate the top

with mushroom slices. Bake for 40 minutes or until set. Let rest for 5 minutes before slicing.

PER SERVING Calories: 191   Fat: 5 g
             Saturated fat: under 1 g   Fiber: 2 g
             Cholesterol: 12 g   Sodium: 428 g
             Calcium: 102 mg   Iron: 3 mg
RESOURCE: Judith Eaton and Karen Lefkowitz

Athenian Tofu

Serves 4

8 ounces orzo or other small pasta

2 cans (1 pound each) whole plum tomatoes, preferably low-salt

2 garlic cloves, chopped

1 teaspoon dried parsley, or 1 tablespoon fresh

1 teaspoon dried basil, or 1 tablespoon fresh

1 teaspoon dried oregano

1 package (10½ ounces) extra-firm low-fat tofu, crumbled

4 ounces feta cheese, crumbled

2 teaspoons capers, rinsed (optional)

1. Cook the orzo according to package directions. Keep hot.

2. Empty the canned tomatoes into a saucepan and bring to a boil, using a large spoon to cut tomatoes into smaller pieces.

3. Add the garlic, parsley, basil, oregano, and tofu. Reduce the heat and simmer for 10 minutes.

4. Add the feta cheese and capers. Simmer for 5 minutes and serve over hot orzo.

PER SERVING   Calories: 365   Fat: 8 g
(EXCLUDING   Saturated fat: 4.5 g   Fiber: 1.5 g
CAPERS)   Cholesterol: 25 g   Sodium: 414 mg
              Calcium: 230 mg   Iron: 4.5 mg
RESOURCE: Judith Eaton and Karen Lefkowitz

Okara Patties with Spicy Peanut Sauce

Serves 8

½ cup diced onion
1 garlic clove, crushed
¼ cup natural-style peanut butter
1 tablespoon honey
2 tablespoons lemon juice
½ teaspoon diced fresh ginger
Dash of cayenne pepper
1 tablespoon vinegar
1 cup water
1 tablespoon low-sodium soy sauce
2 packages (4 patties each) Natural Touch okara patty
4 cups shredded green cabbage
1 cup shredded carrot

1. Coat a large skillet with nonstick cooking spray, then sauté the onion until tender, about 5 minutes.

2. Add the garlic, peanut butter, honey, lemon juice, ginger, cayenne, vinegar, water, and soy sauce. Heat until boiling, and then reduce to a simmer.

3. Heat the okara patties according to package instructions.

4. Steam the cabbage and carrot in separate pans until tender.

5. Serve patties on a bed of the steamed vegetables, and pour sauce over top.

PER SERVING   Calories: 235   Fat: 14 g
              Saturated fat: less than 1 g   Fiber: 2 g
              Cholesterol: 24 mg   Sodium: 460 mg
              Calcium: 31 mg   Iron: less than 1 mg
RESOURCE: Worthington Foods, Inc.

Okara Pattie Foo Yong

Serves 4

1 package (4 patties) Natural Touch okara patty
1 teaspoon cornstarch
1 teaspoon sugar
1 teaspoon vinegar
1 tablespoon low-sodium soy sauce
½ cup water

1. Prepare the patties according to package directions.

2. Combine the ingredients for the sauce in a small saucepan. Cook over medium heat, stirring constantly, until the mixture thickens and boils.

3. Serve over the patties.

PER SERVING   Calories: 169   Fat: 10 g
              Saturated fat: less than 1 g   Fiber: less than 1 g
              Cholesterol: 0   Sodium: 521 mg
              Calcium: 1.4 mg   Iron: less than 1 mg
RESOURCE: Worthington Foods, Inc.

Tempeh Pizza

Serves 2

8 ounces tempeh
1 small onion, chopped
½ red bell pepper, chopped
½ cup sliced fresh mushrooms
½ teaspoon dry Italian seasoning
½ teaspoon dried basil
Salt and pepper to taste
½ cup meatless spaghetti sauce
2 ounces reduced-fat mozzarella cheese

1. Preheat the oven to 450° F.

2. Steam the tempeh for 15 minutes.

3. Coat a large skillet with nonstick cooking spray, and saute the onion and red pepper until onion is translucent, about 3 minutes.

4. Add the mushrooms and seasoning to the skillet, and continue cooking until the mushrooms are tender, stirring frequently, about 3 minutes.

5. Cut tempeh in half and place on baking sheet. Cover each piece with ¼ cup sauce, then half the vegetable mixture. Top each pizza with cheese.

6. Bake for 5 minutes or until the cheese is melted, or microwave on high until cheese is melted.

PER SERVING Calories: 335   Fat: 15 g
              Saturated fat: 1 g   Fiber: 5.5 g
              Cholesterol: 20 g   Sodium: 475 mg
              Calcium: 122 mg   Iron: 3 mg
RESOURCE: Judith Eaton and Karen Lefkowitz

Busy Day Chili

Serves 6

2 cups texturized vegetable protein (TVP) with enough hot
    water to cover (about 1¾ cups)

1 onion, coarsely chopped

1 (15½ ounce) can kidney beans, rinsed and drained

1 cup canned corn

¼ cup chopped fresh parsley

3–4 tablespoons chili powder

3 teaspoons garlic powder

⅓ cup catsup

1 teaspoon low-sodium soy sauce

⅔ cup salsa or picante sauce

2½ cups water

½ cup shredded reduced-fat taco cheese

1. Cover the TVP with hot water and soak until moistened.

2. Coat a large, deep skillet with nonstick cooking spray and sauté the onion until lightly browned, about 5 minutes.

3. Add the TVP and the remainder of ingredients to the skillet. Adjust the seasonings to taste, and simmer the chili for at least 15 minutes to blend the flavors.

PER SERVING Calories: 270   Fat: 4.5 g
                 Saturated fat: under 1 g   Fiber: 14 g
                 Cholesterol: 11 mg   Sodium: 994 mg
                 Calcium: 153 mg   Iron: 5.5 mg
RESOURCE: Judith Eaton and Karen Lefkowitz

Sweet-and-Sour Hawaiian Tempeh

Serves 4

1 package (8 ounces) Lightlife Soy or Three Grain tempeh
1 teaspoon sesame or canola oil
2 carrots, sliced thin
1 cup unsweetened pineapple juice
3 tablespoons low-sodium soy sauce
2 garlic cloves, minced
2 teaspoons grated fresh ginger
1 tablespoon rice wine vinegar
1 tablespoon honey
1 medium red bell pepper, julienned
1 medium green bell pepper, julienned
1 cup broccoli florets, cooked
1 can (8 ounces) unsweetened pineapple chunks
2 teaspoons cornstarch dissolved in ¼ cup water
¼ cup slivered almonds

1. Steam the tempeh for 15 minutes.

2. Cut tempeh into eight 1½-inch squares. Cut each square in half to form 16 triangles, then slice each triangle crosswise so it is ¼-inch thick.

3. Heat the oil in a nonstick skillet and sauté the tempeh pieces for about 5 minutes on each side.

4. Add the carrots, pineapple juice, soy sauce, garlic, and ginger to the skillet. Simmer, covered, over low heat for 10 to 15 minutes.

5. Add the vinegar, honey, peppers, broccoli, and pineapple. Simmer, covered, for 5 minutes.

6. Add the cornstarch mixture and cook 1 minute longer.

7. Serve over steamed rice or noodles. Garnish with almonds.

PER SERVING Calories: 292   Fat: 6 g
             Saturated fat: under 1 g   Fiber: 5 g
             Cholesterol: 0   Sodium: 840 mg
             Calcium: 78 mg   Iron: 2 mg
RESOURCE: Judith Eaton and Karen Lefkowitz

Quick-and-Easy Spinach Lasagna

Serves 5

1 cup texturized vegetable protein (TVP) and hot water to cover (about ⅞ cup)

3 cups prepared fat-free, meatless, low-salt spaghetti sauce or 3 cups homemade sauce

1 container (15 ounces) fat-free ricotta cheese

1 package (10 ounces) frozen chopped spinach, defrosted and squeezed dry.

¼ cup plus 2 tablespoons grated fat-free Parmesan cheese alternative

½ teaspoon dried oregano

2 egg whites

6 no-boil lasagna noodles, or regular lasagna noodles pre-cooked and drained

1¼ cups shredded fat-free mozzarella cheese alternative or reduced-fat soy cheese

1. Preheat the oven to 350° F.

2. Cover the TVP with hot water and soak until moistened, then mix TVP with spaghetti sauce.

3. Mix the ricotta cheese, spinach, ¼ cup Parmesan cheese, oregano, and egg whites.

4. Spread a layer of sauce (about 1 cup) on the bottom of an 8-inch square pan. Place 2 noodles on the sauce, making sure that they do not touch the edges of the pan. Cover the noodles with more sauce, half the spinach mixture, and half the mozzarella. Repeat a layer of noodles, sauce, spinach, and cheese. End with a layer of noodles and sauce. Top with 2 tablespoons of Parmesan cheese.

5. Cover dish with foil and bake for 30 minutes. Uncover and bake for 10 more minutes. Let stand 5 minutes before serving.

PER SERVING Calories: 314   Fat: 2 g
            Saturated fat: under 1 g   Fiber: 4.5 g
            Cholesterol: 20 mg   Sodium: 838 mg
            Calcium: 640 mg   Iron: 5 mg
RESOURCE: Judith Eaton and Karen Lefkowitz

Tempeh Reuben Sandwiches

Serves 4

8 ounces tempeh
¼ cup low-sodium soy sauce
8 slices rye bread
4 teaspoons prepared mustard
1½ cups sauerkraut, drained
4 ounces (4 slices) reduced-fat Swiss cheese

1. Slice the tempeh into quarters and cut each horizontally to make thin slices.

2. In a nonstick skillet, heat 2 tablespoons of the soy sauce and cook the tempeh on one side until brown, about 2 minutes. Add the remaining soy sauce, turn the tempeh, and cook over medium heat until lightly browned, another 2 minutes.

3. Toast the rye bread.

4. Spread mustard on each slice. Top bread with tempeh slice, sauerkraut, and Swiss cheese. Heat on high in microwave until the cheese has melted, about 1½ minutes.

PER SERVING Calories: 362   Fat: 12 g
             Saturated fat: under 1 g   Fiber: 4 g
             Cholesterol: 15 mg   Sodium: 1825 mg
             Calcium: 132 mg   Iron: 4.5 mg
RESOURCE: Judith Eaton and Karen Lefkowitz

Barbecued Tofu

Serves 4

1 pound firm tofu, frozen and then defrosted
2 large onions, thinly sliced
1 cup barbecue sauce, preferably low-fat, low-sodium

1. Squeeze any excess water from the tofu. Slice the block of tofu across its short end into ¼-inch slices.

2. Place the onions in a baking dish and pour ¼ cup of barbecue sauce over them. Add the tofu and the remaining barbecue sauce. Let the tofu and sauce marinate in the refrigerator for several hours.

3. Preheat the oven to 375° F. Bake the tofu and onions for 20 to 30 minutes until the sauce is bubbling hot. (The tofu can also be cooked on the grill, brushing frequently with barbecue sauce.)

4. Serve over rice or stuffed into pieces of crusty French bread.

PER SERVING   Calories: 195   Fat: 6.4 g
              Saturated fat: 2 g   Fiber: 1.7 g
              Cholesterol: 0   Sodium: 240 mg
              Calcium: 35 mg   Iron: 1.6 mg

RESOURCE: Developed by the Soyfoods Association of America with funding from the United Soybean Board

Tofu with Condiments

This makes a great lunch or cold supper!

Serves 2

1 package (10½ ounces) firm or extra firm low-fat tofu
3 scallions
¼ cup chopped fresh cilantro
¼ red bell pepper
1 teaspoon roasted sesame seeds
¼ cup low-sodium soy sauce

1. Drain the tofu. Cut in half on the diagonal to form 2 triangles, then cut a pocket in each triangle.

2. Chop the scallion, cilantro, and pepper finely. Combine with sesame seeds.

3. Stuff half the scallion mixture in each piece of tofu.

4. Pour soy sauce over tofu pockets and marinate in refrigerator for 10 minutes before serving.

PER SERVING Calories: 83   Fat: 2 g
                       Saturated fat: under 1 g   Fiber: under 1 g
                       Cholesterol: 0   Sodium: 743 mg
                       Calcium: 52 mg   Iron: 11 mg
RESOURCE: Judith Eaton and Karen Lefkowitz

Sesame Tofu

Serves 2

¼ cup low-sodium soy sauce
2 tablespoons water
1 tablespoon vinegar
½ teaspoon sugar
½ teaspoon roasted sesame oil
1 scallion, chopped
½ teaspoon finely chopped fresh ginger
1 package (10½ ounces) extra-firm low-fat tofu
1 tablespoon sesame seeds

1. Mix the soy sauce, water, vinegar, sugar, sesame oil, scallion, and ginger in a bowl.

2. Cut the tofu in half horizontally and slice again into 4 pieces.

3. Pour the marinade over the tofu and refrigerate for at least 1 hour.

4. Preheat the oven to 450° F. Spray a baking sheet with non-stick cooking spray.

5. In a dry frying pan, roast the sesame seeds until lightly browned, a few seconds. Press seeds into the tofu and bake for 8 to 10 minutes or until lightly browned.

PER SERVING Calories: 90   Fat: 4 g
             Saturated fat: under 1 g   Fiber: under 1 g
             Cholesterol: 0   Sodium: 455 mg
             Calcium: 39 mg   Iron: 11 mg
RESOURCE: Judith Eaton and Karen Lefkowitz

Noodle Pudding

Serves 9

1 package (10½ ounces) soft low-fat tofu, mashed
½ cup sugar
1 cup raisins
½ cup low-fat cottage cheese
½ cup nonfat sour cream
¼ cup skim milk or low-fat soy milk
1 teaspoon vanilla extract
1 cup canned, crushed unsweetened pineapple in juice, drained
½ cup egg substitute or 4 egg whites
1¼ teaspoons ground cinnamon
3 cups cooked cholesterol-free noodles or regular egg noodles
    (about 6 ounces dry)
¾ cups cornflake crumbs
2 tablespoons brown sugar

1. Preheat the oven to 350°F.

2. In a large bowl, combine the tofu, sugar, raisins, cottage cheese, sour cream, milk, vanilla, pineapple, egg substitute or egg whites, and ½ teaspoon cinnamon; stir well. Gently mix in noodles.

3. Spray an 8- or 9-inch square pan with nonstick cooking spray. Pour mixture into pan.

4. In a small bowl, mix cornflake crumbs, brown sugar, and ¾ teaspoon cinnamon. Spread evenly over the noodle mixture.

5. Bake for 1 hour or until set. Let stand 10 minutes before serving.

PER SERVING Calories: 266   Fat: 1.6 g
            Saturated fat: under 1 g   Fiber: 1 g
            Cholesterol: under 1 g   Sodium: 196 mg
            Calcium: 63 mg   Iron: 4 mg
RESOURCE: Judith Eaton and Karen Lefkowitz

Tempeh-Lemon Broil

Serves 4

1 pound tempeh
1 large onion, sliced
Juice of 3 lemons
¼ cup olive oil
3 tablespoons low-sodium soy sauce
2 garlic cloves, minced

1. Cut the tempeh into 16 chunks. Place in a bowl with the sliced onion.

2. Mix the lemon juice, olive oil, soy sauce, and garlic. Pour mixture over tempeh and onion. Marinate for at least 3 hours in the refrigerator.

3. Preheat the oven to 400° F. Bake for 30 minutes in a roasting pan, basting with the marinade occasionally.

PER SERVING Calories: 223   Fat: 15 g
            Saturated fat: 1 g   Fiber: 3 g
            Cholesterol: 0   Sodium: 307 mg
            Calcium: 63 mg   Iron: 2 mg
RESOURCE: Developed by the Soyfoods Association of America
with funding by the United Soybean Board

Barbecued Grilled Tempeh with Onions

Serves 2

8 ounces tempeh
2 medium onions, thinly sliced
1 cup barbecue sauce, preferably low-fat, low-sodium

1. Preheat the oven to 350° F.

2. Cut the tempeh into 20 cubes.

3. Place the tempeh, onion slices, and barbecue sauce in a casserole sprayed with nonstick cooking spray. Cover and bake for 30 minutes. (The tempeh and onions can also be marinated in the barbecue sauce and then cooked on a grill.)

PER SERVING Calories: 330   Fat: 9 g
             Saturated fat: 0   Fiber: 5 g
             Cholesterol: 0   Sodium: 1170 mg
             Calcium: 95 mg   Iron: 2 mg
RESOURCE: Developed by the Soyfoods Association of America with funding from the United Soybean Board

Tex-Mex Tempeh

A spicy filling for tacos, burritos, or tortillas.

Serves 4

1 package (8 ounces) Lightlife Corn-Jalapeño or Soy tempeh (see Note)

2 tablespoons canola oil

1 medium Spanish onion, in ½-inch cubes

2 garlic cloves, minced

1 teaspoon seeded and minced fresh chili pepper

1 teaspoon sea salt

1½ teaspoons ground cumin

1 tablespoon dried oregano

¼ teaspoon ground nutmeg

2 tablespoons tamari

1 tablespoon brown rice syrup

4 tablespoons tomato paste mixed with 1½–2 cups water

1. Grate or crumble the tempeh. Heat in a skillet and brown the tempeh for 2 minutes. Set aside.

2. In the same skillet, sauté the onion, garlic, chili pepper, and sea salt until onion is translucent, about 3 minutes.

3. Add the tempeh, cumin, oregano, nutmeg, tamari, sweetener, and tomato paste dissolved in water. Stir, cover, and gently simmer until liquid has evaporated, around 10 minutes.

4. Serve with burritos, tortillas, or taco shells.* Garnish with shredded lettuce, sliced tomatoes, avocado, olives, and cilantro.

Note: If using soy tempeh, use 3 garlic cloves, 1 whole fresh chili pepper, 2 teaspoons cumin, and ¼ cup each diced sweet red pepper and corn kernels.

PER SERVING Calories: 206   Fat: 12 g
         Saturated fat: less than 1 g   Fiber: 3 g
         Cholesterol: 0   Sodium: 1174 mg
         Calcium: 87 mg   Iron: 3 mg
RESOURCE: Lynne Paterson, Lightlife Tempeh
* not included in analysis.

Rice and Tofu Loaf

Serves 4

½ pound firm tofu
1½ cups cooked brown rice
1½ tablespoons sesame oil
1 small onion, finely chopped
2 garlic cloves, minced
1 leek, cut in half lengthwise and diced
2 carrots, grated
¼ teaspoon Herbamare seasoning
2 teaspoons dried herbs (thyme, basil, etc.)
1 tablespoon low-sodium soy sauce
Handful of minced fresh parsley

1. Preheat the oven to 375° F.

2. Mash the tofu in a bowl.

3. Heat the oil in a skillet and sauté the onion, garlic, and leek until soft, about 3 minutes. Add Herbamare and dried herbs. Then stir in the carrots and continue to sauté for a few minutes until the vegetables soften.

4. Add the vegetables and remaining ingredients to tofu and mix well.

5. Transfer mixture to an 8½ x 4½-inch loaf pan or casserole dish that has been coated with nonstick cooking spray. Cover with foil and bake for 30 minutes.

6. Remove foil from loaf and bake for another 15 minutes, until the top becomes golden brown and slightly crisp. Allow to cool for about 20 minutes before removing from the pan and slicing.

PER SERVING	Calories: 200	Fat: 8 g
(ANALYZED	Saturated fat: 1 g	Fiber: 1 g
WITHOUT	Cholesterol: 0	Sodium: 270 mg
HERBAMARE)	Calcium: 109 mg	Iron: 5 mg

RESOURCE: Ana McIntyre

Tofu and Mushrooms

This makes a wonderful side dish as well as a main course.

Serves 4

1 can (14 ounces) clear beef broth, preferably low-fat, low-salt

½ cup dry red wine

3 tablespoons low-sodium Kikkoman soy sauce

2 tablespoons sugar

½ pound bite-size fresh mushrooms

1 package (14 or 16 ounces) firm tofu, cut in 1-inch cubes and drained

1½ tablespoons cornstarch

3 scallions, including tops, cut in 2-inch lengths

1. Set aside 2 tablespoons broth. In a large skillet, combine the remaining broth with wine, soy sauce, and sugar. Place in a saucepan and bring to a boil.

2. Add the mushrooms, reduce heat, and cover. Cook for 5 minutes.

3. Add the tofu, cover, and cook for 3 minutes.

4. Dissolve the cornstarch in the reserved broth, then add cornstarch mixture and scallions to the tofu mixture.

5. Cook, stirring gently, until thickened and translucent.

PER SERVING   Calories: 250   Fat: 10 g
              Saturated fat: 2 g   Fiber: 2 g
              Cholesterol: 0   Sodium: 830 mg
              Calcium: 248 mg   Iron: 13 mg
RESOURCE: Azumaya Inc.

Tofu Rice Stir-Fry

Serves 2

1 package (10½ ounces) extra-firm low-fat tofu, drained
     and cut into ½-inch cubes
¼ cup low-sodium soy sauce
¼ cup rice wine vinegar
1 tablespoon sesame oil
1 cup shredded carrots
1 cup sliced celery
½ cup sliced scallions
¼ cup sliced fresh ginger
1 cup cooked white rice

1. Combine the tofu, soy sauce, vinegar, and sesame oil. Marinate in refrigerator for a minimum of 1 hour.

2. Heat all the marinated ingredients in a wok. Add the carrots, celery and ginger. Stir-fry until vegetables are tender but still crisp, about 5 minutes.

3. Add the rice and stir-fry to heat through. Serve hot.

PER SERVING Calories: 337   Fat: 11 g
             Saturated fat: 1 g   Fiber: 5 g
             Cholesterol: 0   Sodium: 1250 mg
             Calcium: 140 mg   Iron: 4 mg
RESOURCE: Mori-nu

Tofu Bouillabaisse

Serves 6

1 pound (16 ounces) firm tofu, drained
1 onion, chopped
1 large garlic clove, minced
2 tablespoons vegetable oil
½ pound white fish fillets (cod, scrod), cubed
1 can (4½ ounces) shrimp, rinsed and drained
1 can (12 ounces) or 1½ bottles (8 ounces each) clam juice
1 can (10¾ ounces) condensed chicken broth
½ cup dry white wine
1 large or 2 small tomatoes, chopped
⅓ cup chopped scallions
¾ teaspoon dried thyme
¼ teaspoon crumbled dried rosemary
1 bay leaf
Salt and pepper to taste (optional)

1. Cut the tofu into small cubes.

2. Sauté the onion and garlic in the oil in large saucepan until soft, about 3 minutes.

3. Add the fish and cook for 5 minutes.

4. Stir in the tofu and remaining ingredients, bring to boil, then simmer for 10 minutes to blend flavors.

PER SERVING   Calories: 264   Fat: 12 g
              Saturated fat: 2 g   Fiber: 54 mg
              Cholesterol: 54 mg   Sodium: 663 mg
              Calcium: 178 mg   Iron: 9 mg
RESOURCE: Azumaya Inc.

Chicken Tetrazzini

Serves 6

2⅓ cups canned low-salt chicken broth

2 packages (10½ ounces each) soft low-fat tofu

¼ cup neufchatel cheese

3 cups sliced fresh mushrooms

½ cup minced onion

1 tablespoon all-purpose flour

¼ cup grated Parmesan cheese, preferably fat-free cheese
    alternative

¼ cup dry sherry

¼ teaspoon salt

1½ teaspoons garlic powder

½ teaspoon black pepper

1½ cups frozen peas

1 jar (2 ounces) pimiento, drained and diced

½ pound spaghetti

2 cups chopped cooked chicken breast (about ½ pound)

1 teaspoon Worcestershire sauce

1. Preheat the oven to 350° F.

2. In food processor, mix the chicken broth, tofu, and Neuf-chatel cheese until smooth. Set aside.

3. Spray a large skillet with nonstick cooking spray. Sauté the mushrooms and onion over medium heat for 6 minutes.

4. Stir the flour into the mushroom mixture. Gradually add the tofu mixture. Bring to a boil and cook 5 minutes, stirring constantly.

5. Remove skillet from heat and stir in 2 tablespoons Parmesan cheese, sherry, salt, garlic powder, and pepper. Stir, add the peas and pimiento, then set aside.

6. Break the spaghetti into 4 lengths and cook according to package directions. Drain.

7. Stir spaghetti and chicken into the tofu mixture. Mix in the Worcestershire sauce, then pour into a 3-quart casserole coated with nonstick cooking spray. Sprinkle top with remaining Parmesan cheese.

8. Cover the casserole and bake for 20 minutes, then uncover and bake an additional 10 minutes. Let stand 5 minutes before serving.

PER SERVING Calories: 302   Fat: 7 g
             Saturated fat: 2 g   Fiber: 3 g
             Cholesterol: 32 mg   Sodium: 233 mg
             Calcium: 97 mg   Iron: 25 mg
RESOURCE: Judith Eaton and Karen Lefkowitz

Chicken and Tofu Stir-Fry

Serves 6

1 pound extra-firm tofu, drained and cut in ¾-inch cubes
¼ cup low-sodium soy sauce
1 tablespoon cornstarch
1 whole chicken breast, skinned, boned, and cut into thin
    strips
1 tablespoon canola oil
½ pound broccoli, chopped
1 onion, cut into wedges
1 cup bean sprouts
2 garlic cloves, halved
6 cups cooked brown rice

1. Marinate the tofu in 2 tablespoons of the soy sauce for 10 minutes. Drain well.

2. Combine the used soy sauce with the cornstarch and marinate the chicken for 15 minutes.

3. In a large skillet or wok, stir-fry the tofu for 2 minutes in the oil until light brown (if using a wok, heat before adding oil).

4. Remove tofu and stir-fry the broccoli for 3 minutes. Add the onion and stir-fry 2 more minutes. Add the bean sprouts and stir-fry 1 minute.

5. Remove all the vegetables from the skillet or wok. Add more oil if necessary and toss in the garlic, stir-frying for 1 minute. Discard garlic and add chicken and marinade. Cook 2 to 3 minutes. Add remaining 2 tablespoons soy sauce, vegetables, and tofu; heat thoroughly.

6. Serve with cooked brown rice.

PER SERVING Calories: 367   Fat: 7 g
             Saturated fat: 1 g   Fiber: 5 g
             Cholesterol: 24 mg   Sodium: 483 mg
             Calcium: 80 mg   Iron: 3 mg

RESOURCE: Adapted from a recipe developed by Bountiful Bean Soyfoods

Chicken Paprika

Serves 4

½ pound noodles, preferably no-yolks pasta

1 teaspoon canola oil

1 cup chopped onion

2 tablespoons Hungarian paprika

1½ cups fat-free, low-salt chicken broth

½ cup dry sherry

1 pound boneless and skinless chicken breast, cut into cubes

1 package (10½ ounces) firm low-fat tofu

1 tablespoon all-purpose flour

1. Cook the noodles according to package directions.

2. In a large, nonstick skillet, heat the oil, add the onions, and cook until lightly browned.

3. Add the paprika and cook for another minute. Add the chicken broth and sherry, then bring to a boil over high heat. Add the chicken cubes and cook over medium heat for 30 minutes.

4. Puree the tofu with the flour in a blender or food processor. Add to the skillet and bring to a boil. Serve over noodles.

PER SERVING Calories: 495   Fat: 12.5 g
             Saturated fat: 2.5 g   Fiber: under 1 g
             Cholesterol: 94 mg   Sodium: 264 mg
             Calcium: 56 mg   Iron: 4.5 mg
RESOURCE: Judith Eaton and Karen Lefkowitz

Beefy Tofu Enchiladas

Serves 8

1 package (10½ ounces) firm tofu, mashed
½ cup chopped onion
1 pound extra-lean ground beef, browned and drained
1 can (4 ounces) chopped green chilies
1 garlic clove, minced
1 teaspoon dried cilantro
½ teaspoon cumin seed
2 cups drained and diced tomatoes
8 8-inch flour tortillas
2 cups thick tomato salsa
*1 cup shredded cheddar cheese, preferably reduced-fat, low-
  salt*

1. Preheat the oven to 350° F. Lightly spray a 9 x 13-inch baking dish with nonstick cooking spray.

2. In a bowl, combine all the ingredients except the tortillas, salsa, and cheese.

3. Place ½ cup of the mixture in the center of each tortilla and roll up. Place in the baking dish, seam side down.

4. Pour the salsa over the enchiladas. Sprinkle with shredded cheese. Cover pan with aluminum foil and bake for 25 to 30 minutes.

PER SERVING Calories: 370   Fat: 17 g
             Saturated fat: 4.5 g   Fiber: 1 g
             Cholesterol: 50 mg   Sodium: 600 mg
             Calcium: 290 mg   Iron: 4 mg
RESOURCE: Soy Ohio

Meat Loaf

Serves 4

½ pound extra-lean ground beef
½ pound extra-firm low-fat tofu, mashed
½ cup bread crumbs, preferably from whole wheat bread
½ package dry onion soup mix
2 egg whites
1 carrot, grated
1 can (8 ounces) tomato sauce, preferably low-salt

1. Preheat the oven to 350° F.

2. In a bowl, mix the beef, tofu, bread crumbs, soup mix, egg whites, and carrot with ½ can tomato sauce.

3. On a broiler pan (or use a loaf pan [8½ x 4½-inch]), shape the mixture into a loaf. Top with remaining tomato sauce and bake for 1 hour or until cooked through.

PER SERVING Calories: 265   Fat: 10 g
             Saturated fat: 4 g   Fiber: 1 g
             Cholesterol: 60 mg   Sodium: 261 mg
             Calcium: 60 mg   Iron: 9 mg
RESOURCE: Judith Eaton and Karen Lefkowitz

Breads and Breakfasts

Peach Breakfast Soufflé

Serves 4

1 package (8.4 ounces) Creamy Original Vitasoy soy milk
1 large egg and 1 egg white
1 teaspoon orange juice concentrate
1 teaspoon honey or maple syrup
½ teaspoon each grated lemon and orange zest
¼ teaspoon ground cinnamon
2 large slices whole-grain bread
2 fresh peaches, 1 chopped and 1 sliced

1. Preheat the oven to 375° F. Coat a small 2-quart casserole with nonstick cooking spray.

2. Beat together all the ingredients except the bread and sliced peach.

3. Lay one slice of bread in the casserole and pour half the liquid over it. Top with half the sliced peaches, then the other slice of bread. Cover with the remaining liquid and finally with the remaining sliced peaches.

4. Bake for 60 minutes or until the top is golden and firm to the touch. Let cool before serving.

PER SERVING Calories: 107   Fat: 3g
             Saturated fat: less than 1g   Fiber: 1g
             Cholesterol: 53 mg   Sodium: 93 mg
             Calcium: 43 mg   Iron: 1 mg
RESOURCE: Vitasoy, Inc.

Tolffins

Makes 12 muffins

1 cup old-fashioned rolled oats
¾ cup whole wheat pastry flour
¼ cup soy flour, preferably defatted
2 teaspoons baking powder
½ teaspoon salt
1 teaspoon ground cinnamon
¼ teaspoon ground cloves
½ cup chopped walnuts
½ cup raisins
1 large apple, chopped
¼ cup banana, mashed
¼ cup maple syrup
1 package (10½ ounces) soft low-fat tofu

1. Preheat oven to 350° F. Spray a muffin tin with nonstick cooking spray.

2. Combine the oats, flours, baking powder, salt, cinnamon, cloves, walnuts, raisins, and apple.

3. Process the banana, maple syrup, and tofu in a food processor until completely blended.

4. Combine the tofu mixture with the dry ingredients until moistened. Pour into muffin cups and bake for 35 to 45 minutes, or until a toothpick inserted in center comes out clean. Cool completely before eating.

PER SERVING: Calories: 158   Fat: 5 g
              Saturated fat: under 1 g   Fiber: 2 g
              Cholesterol: 0   Sodium: 153 mg
              Calcium: 83 mg   Iron: 1 mg
RESOURCE: Judith Eaton and Karen Lefkowitz

Zucchini Bread

Makes 2 loaves of bread (about 13 slices each)

1 cup all-purpose flour
1¼ cups whole wheat flour
¾ cup soy flour, preferably defatted
2 teaspoons ground cinnamon
1 teaspoon baking powder
1 teaspoon baking soda
1 cup raisins
½ cup egg substitute or 4 egg whites
⅓ cup unsweetened applesauce
1 package (10½ ounces) soft low-fat tofu, pureed
1 cup packed brown sugar
2 teaspoons vanilla extract
2 cups finely shredded zucchini

1. Preheat the oven to 350° F. Coat two 8 x 4-inch loaf pans with nonstick spray.

2. Combine the flours, cinnamon, baking powder, baking soda, and raisins in a bowl.

3. In a large bowl, beat the egg substitute or egg whites until foamy. Combine eggs with applesauce, tofu, brown sugar, and vanilla. Stir in zucchini.

4. Add the flour mixture and mix until well blended.

5. Pour batter into prepared pans and bake for 55 minutes or until a toothpick inserted in center comes out clean.

6. Cool pans on a rack for 10 minutes. Remove loaves from pans and cool thoroughly before slicing.

PER SERVING (1 SLICE)		
Calories: 113		Fat: 1 g
Saturated fat: under 1 g		Fiber: 1 g
Cholesterol: 0		Sodium: 61 mg
Calcium: 27 mg		Iron: 1 mg

RESOURCE: Judith Eaton and Karen Lefkowitz

Eastern Omelet

This simple omelet can easily be dressed up with the addition of sliced mushrooms, peas, chopped spinach, or bean sprouts.

Serves 4

1 cup drained diced Azumaya Kinugosihi soft tofu
10 egg whites, beaten
⅓ cup low-fat milk
3 tablespoons chopped scallion
½ teaspoon salt
⅛ teaspoon pepper
1 tablespoon butter or margarine or nonstick cooking spray
Soy sauce or light tamari to taste (optional)

1. Combine the tofu, egg whites, milk, scallion, salt, and pepper in a bowl.

2. Melt the butter or shortening in a large skillet or coat with nonstick cooking spray.

3. Add the egg-tofu mixture and cook slowly. Run a spatula around the edge, lifting to allow any uncooked portion to flow underneath. When the eggs are set, fold in half and turn out onto a warmed serving platter. Serve with soy sauce if desired.

PER SERVING Calories: 112   Fat: 5 g
             Saturated fat: 1 g   Fiber: 1 g
             Cholesterol: 0   Sodium: 419 mg
             Calcium: 55 mg   Iron: 1 mg
RESOURCE: Adapted from a recipe developed by Azumaya Inc.

Apple Pancakes

Serves 4; makes 12 pancakes

3 tablespoons sugar

½ teaspoon ground cinnamon

¼ teaspoon ground nutmeg

⅛ teaspoon salt

1 cup all-purpose flour

1 tablespoon soy flour

2 teaspoons baking powder

¾ cup soy milk

1 teaspoon vanilla extract

2 tablespoons margarine, melted and cooled

1 tart apple, peeled, cored, and grated

1. Mix the sugar with the cinnamon, nutmeg, and salt. Blend sugar mixture with the flours and baking soda.

2. In a separate bowl, whisk together the soy milk, vanilla, and margarine. Pour over the dry mixture and blend well. Fold in the apples.

3. Pour ¼ cup of batter onto a hot nonstick griddle or pan. Cook for about 2 minutes on one side, or until bubbles appear on surface, then flip and cook for another minute or until heated through.

4. Serve topped with applesauce and maple syrup.

PER SERVING	Calories: 80	Fat: 2 g
(PER PANCAKE)	Saturated fat: less than 1 g	Fiber: less than 1 g
	Cholesterol: 0	Sodium: 85 mg
	Calcium: 60 mg	Iron: less than 1 mg

RESOURCE: Developed by the Soyfoods Association of America
with funding from the United Soybean Board

Banana Pancakes

Serves 4

1 cup all-purpose flour
½ cup soy flour, preferably defatted
1 teaspoon salt
1¾ teaspoons baking powder
3 tablespoons soybean oil
1¼ cups plain soy milk
2 bananas, thinly sliced
Fresh, sliced fruit or maple syrup (optional)

1. Sift together the flours, salt, and baking powder.

2. In a separate bowl, mix the oil and milk. Add quickly to the dry ingredients, stirring just to blend. Add the bananas and stir into the batter with just a few strokes.

3. Pour batter by ¼ cupfuls onto a lightly oiled griddle and cook for 2 to 3 minutes or until bubbles begin to form on the pancakes. Then flip and cook on the other side for 1 to 2 minutes. Serve with fresh fruit or maple syrup.

PER SERVING Calories: 363   Fat: 12 g
             Saturated fat: 2g   Fiber: 5 g
             Cholesterol: 0   Sodium: 553 mg
             Calcium: 62 mg   Iron: 3 mg
RESOURCE: United Soybean Board

Desserts

Chocolate Tofu Berry Whip

An unbelievably delicious dessert.

Serves 3

1 package (10½ ounces) firm or extra-firm low-fat tofu
1 cup raspberries or any other berries, frozen and unsweet-
    ened
½ cup fruit-sweetened blackberry jam (14 calories per tea-
    spoon)
1 teaspoon vanilla extract
1 teaspoon fresh lemon juice
1 tablespoon cocoa powder

1. Place the tofu, berries, jam, vanilla, lemon juice,and cocoa powder in a food processor. Process until smooth.

2. Spoon into parfait glasses and serve.

PER SERVING Calories: 182   Fat: 1 g
            Saturated fat: less than 1 g   Fiber: 2 g
            Cholesterol: 0   Sodium: 95 mg
            Calcium: 30 mg.   Iron: 8 mg
RESOURCE: Judith Eaton and Karen Lefkowitz

Chocolate Chip Cookies

Makes approximately 80 cookies

1¾ cups all-purpose flour
¾ cup soy flour, preferably defatted
½ cup Dutch-process cocoa
1 teaspoon baking soda
1 jar (2½ ounces) strained prunes (baby food)
2 teaspoons vanilla extract
2 tablespoons light corn syrup
1 cup granulated sugar
1 cup packed light brown sugar
½ cup soft low-fat tofu
¼ cup skim milk or low-fat soy milk
½ cup miniature chocolate chips

1. Preheat the oven to 350° F. Spray cookie sheets with non-stick cooking spray.

2. In a large bowl, mix the flours, cocoa, and baking soda and set aside.

3. In another bowl, mix the prunes, vanilla, corn syrup, sugars, tofu, and milk. Beat with an electric mixer at high speed until well blended. Add this mixture to the dry mixture and blend well. Add chocolate chips and mix.

4. Drop a teaspoonful of batter at a time onto the cookie sheet, leaving about 1 inch between the cookies. Bake for 10 minutes. Let cool on rack.

PER COOKIE Calories: 45   Fat: under 1 g
            Saturated fat: under 1 g   Fiber: under 1 g
            Cholesterol: under 1 g   Sodium: 18 mg
            Calcium: 7 mg   Iron: under 1 mg
RESOURCE: Judith Eaton and Karen Lefkowitz

Chocolate Cream Pie

Serves 8

PIE CRUST

¼ cup low-fat margarine
1¼ cups graham cracker crumbs

FILLING

1 cup sugar
1 envelope unflavored gelatin
⅓ cup Dutch-process cocoa
¾ cup skim milk or fat-reduced soy milk
1 package (10½ ounces) firm light tofu, pureed
1 teaspoon vanilla extract

1. Melt the margarine, then add to bread crumbs and blend well.

2. Press crumbs into a 9-inch pie pan. Chill at least 15 minutes.

3. In a medium saucepan, mix the sugar, gelatin, and cocoa. Slowly stir in the milk and let stand 5 minutes.

4. Cook over medium heat, stirring constantly, until the mixture comes to a boil and gelatin is dissolved. Add the tofu and vanilla; stir until well combined.

5. Pour into prepared crust and chill several hours until firm.

PER SERVING Calories: 255   Fat: 6 g
             Saturated fat: under 1 g   Fiber: under 1 g
             Cholesterol: under 1 g   Sodium: 200 mg
             Calcium: 50 mg   Iron: 2 mg
RESOURCE: Judith Eaton and Karen Lefkowitz

Tofu Brownies

Gooey and delicious.

Makes 16 brownies

¾ cup all-purpose flour
½ cup soy flour, preferably defatted
⅓ cup Dutch-process cocoa
1¼ cups sugar
¼ teaspoon baking soda
2 tablespoons cornstarch
1 jar (2½ ounces) strained prunes (baby food)
½ cup soft low-fat tofu, pureed
2 teaspoons vanilla extract
2 tablespoons light corn syrup
¼ cup miniature chocolate chips or chopped walnuts (optional)

1. Preheat the oven to 350° F. Coat an 8-inch square pan with nonstick cooking spray.

2. Sift together in a large bowl the flours, cocoa, ½ cup sugar, baking soda, and cornstarch. Mix well.

3. In another bowl, with an electric beater or whisk, mix the prunes, tofu, vanilla, corn syrup, and ¾ cup sugar until well blended.

4. Combine wet ingredients and dry ingredients; mix until smooth. The batter will be very thick. Fold in optional chips or walnuts.

5. Bake for 25 minutes. Cool and cut into 16 squares.

PER SERVING Calories: 120   Fat: under 1 g
             Saturated fat: under 1 g   Fiber: under 1 g
             Cholesterol: 0   Sodium: 24 mg
             Calcium: 10 mg   Iron: 1 mg
RESOURCE: Judith Eaton and Karen Lefkowitz

Tofu Strawberry Cheese Cake

Serves 8

CRUST

1 cup graham cracker crumbs

2 tablespoons canola oil

1 tablespoon brown sugar

FILLING

¾ cup egg substitute

1 package (10½ ounces) extra-firm low-fat tofu, drained and cut into small pieces

¼ cup maple syrup

2 tablespoons lemon juice

1 teaspoon vanilla extract

3 ounces fat-free ricotta cheese

TOPPING

2 cups fresh strawberries
½ cup all-fruit strawberry preserves

1. Preheat the oven to 325° F.

2. Mix the graham cracker crumbs with the oil and brown sugar. Press into a 9-inch pie pan.

3. In a food processor, whip the egg substitute. Add the tofu, syrup, lemon juice, and vanilla. Blend until smooth. Add the ricotta cheese and blend until smooth.

4. Pour filling into pie crust and bake for 45 to 55 minutes. Cool for 5 minutes.

5. Cover pie with fruit. Heat the preserves, then pour over strawberries. Chill for several hours before serving.

PER SERVING Calories: 205 Fat: 5 g
Saturated fat: under 1 g Fiber: under 1 g
Cholesterol: 3 mg Sodium: 160 mg
Calcium: 65 mg Iron: 4 mg
RESOURCE: Judith Eaton and Karen Lefkowitz

Creamy Spritzer

Serves 2

½ cup vanilla-flavored soy milk, preferably low-fat
½ cup orange juice
1 cup sparkling water

1. Blend the soy milk and orange juice in a blender.

2. Pour mixture over ice and add sparkling water.

PER SERVING   Calories: 60   Fat: 12 g
                    Saturated fat: 2 g   Fiber: 0
                    Cholesterol: 0   Sodium: 54 mg
                    Calcium: 60 mg   Iron: 3 mg
RESOURCE: United Soybean Board

Tofu Pumpkin Pie

Serves 8

1 can (16 ounces) pureed pumpkin

¾ cups sugar

½ teaspoon salt

1 teaspoon ground cinnamon

½ teaspoon ground ginger

¼ teaspoon ground cloves

*1 package (10½ ounces) soft tofu processed in a blender until
    smooth*

1 9-inch unbaked pie shell

1. Preheat the oven to 425° F.

2. Cream the pumpkin and sugar. Add the salt, spices, and
tofu, mixing thoroughly.

3. Pour mixture into pie shell and bake for 15 minutes. Lower
the heat to 350° F. and bake for an additional 40 minutes.

4. Chill before serving.

PER SERVING Calories: 195   Fat: 6 g
             Saturated fat: 2 g   Fiber: 2 g
             Cholesterol: 0   Sodium: 240 mg
             Calcium: 35 mg   Iron: 2 mg
RESOURCE: Developed by the Soyfoods Association of America
with funding from the United Soybean Board

Strawberry Fluff

Serves 4

1 package (10½ ounces) soft tofu, drained
3 tablespoons honey
2½ cups frozen strawberries, thawed and drained

1. In blender or food processor, combine the tofu and honey.
Blend until smooth and creamy.

2. Add the strawberries, ½ cup at a time. Allow some berries
to remain in chunks.

3. Pour into stemmed glasses. Chill and serve.

PER SERVING Calories: 125   Fat: 2 g
             Saturated fat: less than 1 g   Fiber: 2 g
             Cholesterol: 0   Sodium: 25 mg
             Calcium: 35 mg   Iron: 1.5 mg
RESOURCE: Missouri Soybean Board

Super-Moist Carrot Cake

Serves 16

2 cups plus 2 tablespoons whole wheat flour

2½ teaspoons ground cinnamon

1½ teaspoons ground nutmeg

1½ teaspoons baking soda

¾ teaspoon ground cloves

1 package (10½ ounces) soft tofu, drained

½ cup vegetable oil

⅔ cup honey

2 teaspoons vanilla extract

2¼ cups finely shredded carrots

1 can (8 ounces) unsweetened crushed pineapple in juice, drained

1. Preheat the oven to 350° F.

2. In a medium bowl, combine the flour, cinnamon, nutmeg, baking soda, and cloves. Set aside.

3. In a food processor or blender, combine the tofu, oil, honey, and vanilla. Blend until smooth.

4. Pour the tofu mixture into the flour mixture. Mix until dry ingredients are moist, then add the carrots and pineapple. Stir until well blended.

5. Pour mixture into an ungreased 8-inch square baking pan. Bake for 40 to 45 minutes or until a toothpick inserted in the center of the cake comes out clean. Serve slightly warm.

PER SERVING Calories: 180   Fat: 8 g
             Saturated fat: 1 g   Fiber: 2.5 g
             Cholesterol: 0   Sodium: 125 mg
             Calcium: 24 mg   Iron: 1.1 mg
RESOURCE: Missouri Soybean Board

Vanilla Pudding

Serves 3

½ cup sugar
2 tablespoons cornstarch
⅛ teaspoon salt
1½ cups plain soy milk
1 teaspoon vanilla extract

1. In a saucepan, stir together the sugar, cornstarch, and salt. Slowly add the soy milk, stirring to prevent lumps.

2. Bring the mixture to boil. Lower heat to a simmer, stirring constantly for about 5 minutes, until mixture is thick and creamy. Remove from heat.

3. Stir in the vanilla and pour into dessert cups. Chill until mixture sets.

PER SERVING Calories: 145   Fat: 2 g
             Saturated fat: less than 1 g   Fiber 1 g
             Cholesterol: 0   Sodium: 78 mg
             Calcium: 4 mg   Iron: Less than 1 mg
RESOURCE: Developed by the Soyfoods Association of America and the United Soybean Advisory Board

"Piña Colada"

Serves 4

1 package (10½ ounces) soft tofu
1½ large ripe bananas
2 cups unsweetened pineapple juice
½ teaspoon coconut extract
2 tablespoons sugar or to taste

1. In a blender or a food processor, combine all the ingredients. Whip until smooth.

2. Cover and chill in the refrigerator for at least 1 hour before serving, or serve over crushed ice.

PER SERVING (ANALYZED WITHOUT COCONUT EXTRACT)		
Calories: 178		Fat: 2.4 g
Saturated fat: less than 1 g		Fiber: 1.6 g
Cholesterol: 0		Sodium: 161 mg
Calcium: 41 mg		Iron: 1 mg

RESOURCE: Mori-nu

Low-Cal Chocolate Mousse

Serves 10

¾ cup honey or fruit sweetener
½ cup cocoa powder
3 teaspoons vanilla
2 packages (10½ ounces each) low-fat firm tofu, drained

1. Heat honey or fruit sweetener for 90 seconds in a microwave. Pour over cocoa powder. Add vanilla. Stir until smooth.

2. Blend tofu until smooth. Add chocolate mixture and continue blending for 1 minute. Chill 1 to 2 hours.

PER SERVING   Calories: 114   Fat: 1 g
              Saturated fat: 0   Fiber 0
              Cholesterol: 0   Sodium: 53 mg
              Calcium: 19 mg   Iron: 1 mg
RESOURCE: Mori-nu

Glossary

Antioxidant   We couldn't live without oxygen, yet every time we breath it in, we are also making ourselves vulnerable to the formation of free radicals—unstable oxygen molecules that can react with healthy cells in harmful ways. Free radicals have been blamed for everything from producing cancerous changes in cells to promoting the formation of plaque deposits in arteries to promoting arthritis and other degenerative diseases often associated with aging. Antioxidants are compounds that work with the body's defense system to prevent damage by free radicals.

Amino acids   These compounds are the building blocks of protein. Some amino acids are produced by the body; others, called *essential amino acids,* must be obtained through food.

Atherosclerosis   This condition occurs when the arteries delivering blood to the heart become clogged with plaque, a waxy, yellowish substance that impedes the flow of blood to the heart.

Bowman-Birk Inhibitor (BBI)   This compound found in soy food is a protease inhibitor—that is, it blocks the action of certain enzymes that can promote the growth of tumors.

Cancer initiator   An initiator produces deleterious changes in cells that can eventually lead to the formation of cancerous growths.

Cancer promoter   A cancer promoter encourages the proliferation of "bad" cells that can promote tumor growth.

Carcinogen Any substance that either initiates or promotes cancer.

Coronary artery disease (CAD) When the coronary arteries delivering blood to the heart become filled with plaque, they can eventually become so narrow that the blood flow to the heart is impaired. If the blood supply to the heart is cut off, a portion of the heart muscle will die, resulting in a heart attack.

Chelator A compound that binds with metals in the body, preventing their absorption. Phytic acid is a chelator in soy that binds with iron and zinc.

Cholesterol A fatlike substance produced by the liver or obtained through food that is essential for the production of cell membranes, sex hormones, and for the production of vitamin D, among other things. High levels of blood cholesterol have been associated with an increased risk of developing CAD.

Daidzein An isoflavone found in soy that has been shown to have anticarcinogenic properties.

Equol An estrogenic compound produced by gut bacteria from isoflavones, found in the urine of people who eat soy.

Estradiol The most common circulating estrogen in premenopausal women.

Estrone The most common circulating estrogen in postmenopausal women.

Genistein An isoflavone found exclusively in soy foods that in laboratory studies has been shown to inhibit the growth of both breast cancer and prostate cancer cells. Genistein has also been shown to convert abnormal cancer cells into normal ones, thus thwarting the spread of cancer.

High-density lipoprotein (HDL) HDL is sometimes called "good cholesterol" because it is the body's major carrier of cholesterol to the liver for excretion in the bile. The ratio between total cholesterol and HDL should not exceed 6:1.

Isolated Soy Protein (ISP) A concentrated soy protein product that contains no less than 90 percent protein.

Isoflavones Compounds found in soy that resemble the natural estrogens produced in the body and are mildly estrogenic. Many of these compounds are believed to protect against cancer.

Low-density lipoprotein (LDL) Sometimes referred to as "bad cholesterol," LDLs carry cholesterol through the bloodstream. Studies show that high levels of LDL enhance the risk of developing CAD.

Legume Legumes are a food group containing dried beans, including soybeans, peas, lentils, and kidney beans.

Lysine An essential amino acid found in soy that is usually missing from food plants.

mg/dl Milligrams per deciliter.

Miso A fermented paste from soybeans that is often used as a soup base.

Okara The pulp from the soybeans that is a by-product of the tofu-making process. Okara can be used in cooking.

Phytic acid A compound found in soy that has been shown to inhibit the growth of tumors in animals.

Phytochemicals Compounds found in food plants that may protect against disease.

Phytoestrogens Plant compounds that are structurally similar to naturally produced estrogen and that bind with estrogen receptors in the body. Phytoestrogens are believed to protect against breast cancer and prostate cancer, two hormone-dependent cancers.

Prostate gland A small walnut-size gland located between the bladder and the penis, above the rectum.

Protein Present in every cell of the body, protein is made up of chains of amino acids. Protein groups also regulate the production of enzymes and hormones.

Protease inhibitors These compounds inhibit the action of certain enzymes that promote the growth of tumors.

Tempeh A fermented soy product with a meaty texture and a nutty flavor that is popular in Indonesia.

Tofu A bean curd produced from soybeans.

Yuba The layer of skin that forms on freshly made soy milk, which can be dried and used in cooking.

Resources

To get a copy of Dr. Mindell's complete program for a healthy life and to subscribe to his newsletter, *Joy of Health,* call 1-800-777-5005.

The following companies or organizations will provide information on soy foods.

General Information

United Soybean Board Hotline
1-800-TALK-SOY
The United Soybean Board will provide information on various soy products as well as recipes. A free videotape on new uses for soybeans is available to business and industry groups.

American Soybean Association
540 Maryville Centre Drive, Suite 390
St. Louis, Missouri 63141
Will provide information on soy foods and recipes.

Archer Daniels Midland (ADM)
Box 1470
Decatur, Illinois 62525
ADM offers a line of burgers made from texturized vegetable protein.

Soyfoods Center
P.O. Box 234
Lafayette, California 94549
510-283-2991
Headed by William Shurtleff and Akiko Aoyagi Shurtleff, co-authors of *The Book of Tofu* and other books on soy foods, the Soyfoods Center offers a wealth of material on soy products for consumers and business groups.

Bountiful Bean Soyfoods
A Vermont West Company
620 Main Street, Box 329
Ridgeway, Wisconsin 53582-0329
Will provide recipe brochure.

Missouri Soybean Merchandising Council
P.O. Box 104778
520 Ellis Boulevard, Suite N
Jefferson City, Missouri 65110
Will provide recipe brochure.

Ohio Soybean Council
P.O. Box 479
Columbus, Ohio 43216-0479
614-249-2492
Will provide a free recipe booklet.

Worthington Foods, Inc.
900 Proprietors Road
Worthington, Ohio 43085
Will provide information on soy analogs and recipes.

Lightlife Foods, Inc.
1-800-274-6001
Will provide recipe brochure.

Information on Tofu

Mori-nu Tofu
1-800-NOW-TOFU
Morinaga, producers of Mori-nu tofu, will ship boxes of its
low-fat and regular, aseptically packaged tofu anywhere in the
United States, packed twenty-four in a case. Mori-nu tofu has
a shelf life of ten months and does not need refrigeration. It
comes in three varieties: Silken Soft, Silken Firm, Silken Extra-
Firm. Morinaga also offers a diet plan—tofu cookbook. Call the

toll-free number for information on how to buy the diet program and videotape.

Reduced Fat Tofu
White Wave Soy Foods
Boulder, Colorado 80301
White Wave tofu is certified organic. To locate the nearest vendor in your area, call 800-488-9283.

Azumaya Inc.
1575 Burke Avenue
San Francisco, California 94124
Offers free recipe brochure

Information on Tempeh

Betsy's Tempeh
S & P Farm
14780 Beardslee Road
Perry, Michigan 48872
517-675-5213
Offers free recipe brochure.

Information on Soy Milk

Healthy Recipes Offer
Eden Foods
701 Tecumseh Road
Clinton, Michigan 49236
Edensoy offers a free soy milk cookbook.

Vitasoy (USA) Inc.
99 Park Lane
Brisbane, California 94005
1-800-VITASOY
Offers recipes and information.

Westbrae Natural Foods (Westsoy Products)
P.O. Box 48006
Gardenia, California 90248
310-886-8200
1-800-SOY-MILK

Information on Soy Protein Isolate

Fearn Natural Foods
Modern Products
Milwaukee, Wisconsin 53209
Send a stamped, self-addressed envelope for a recipe folder
using soy protein isolate

Information on Soy Protein Beverages

Nutritious Foods:
1-800-445-3350
To order Take Care beverage powders and food ingredients.

Nature's Plus
548 Broad Hollow Road
Melville, New York 11747
(516) 293-0030
For information on where to buy Spiru-tein high-protein
shakes.

Selected Bibliography

Adlercreutz, H. "Western Diet and Western Disease: Some Hormonal and Biochemical Mechanisms and Associations." *Scandinavian Journal of Clinical and Laboratory Investigations* 50, Supplement 201(1990):3–23.

———— H., "Ligans and Phytoestrogens: Possible Preventive Roles in Cancer." *Frontiers of Gastrointestinal Research* 14(1988):165–176.

Adlercreutz, H., E. Hämäläinen, S. Gorbach, and B. Goldin. "Dietary Phyto-oestrogens and the Menopause in Japan." *The Lancet* 339 (May 16, 1992):1233.

Adlercreutz, H., H. Markkanen, and S. Watanabe. "Plasma Concentrations of Phyto-oestrogens in Japanese Men." *The Lancet* 342 (November 13, 1993):1209–1210.

Adlercreutz, H., K. Höckerstedt, C. Bannwart, et al. "Effect of Dietary Components, Including Lignans and Phytoestrogens, on Enterohepatic Circulation and Liver Metabolism of Estrogens and on Sex Hormone Binding Globulin (SHBG)." *Journal of Steroid Biochemistry* 27, no. 4–6(1987):1135–1144.

Adlercreutz, H., R. Heikkinen, M. Woods, et al. "Excretion of the Lignans Enterolactone and Enterodiol and of Equol in Omnivorous and Vegetarian Postmenopausal Women and in Women With Breast Cancer." *The Lancet* (December 11, 1982):1295–1299.

Adlercreutz, H., T. Fostis, C. Bannwart, et al. "Determination of Urinary Lignans and Phytoestrogen Metabolites, Potential Antiestrogens and Anticarcinogens in Urine of Women on Various Habitual Diets." *Journal of Steroid Biochemistry* 25, no. 5B(1986):791–797.

Adlercreutz, H., T. Fotsis, K. Höckerstedt, et al. "Diet and Urinary Estrogen Profile in Premenopausal Omnivorous and Vegetarian Women and in Premenopausal Women with Breast Cancer." *Journal of Steroid Biochemistry* 34, no. 1–6(1989):527–530.

Adlercreutz, H., Y. Mousavi, J. Clark, et al. "Dietary phytoestrogens and Cancer: *in Vitro* and *in Vivo* Studies." *Journal of Steroid Biochemistry and Molecular Biology* 41, no. 3–8(1992):331–337.

Adlercreutz, H., Y. Mousavi, and K. Höckerstedt. "Diet and Breast Cancer." *Acta Oncologica* 31, no. 2(1992):175–181.

Akiyama, T., J. Ishida, S. Nakagawa, et al. "Genistein, a Specific Inhibitor of Tyrosine-Specific Protein Kinases." *Journal of Biological Chemistry* 262, no. 12 (April 25, 1987):5592–5595.

Anderson, J. W., N. J. Gustafson, C. A. Bryant, and J. Tietyen-Clark. "Dietary Fiber and Diabetes: A Comprehensive Review and Practical. Application." *Journal of the American Dietetic Association* 87, no. 9(1987):1189–1197.

Armstrong, B. K., J. B. Brown, H. T. Clark, et al. "Diet and Reproductive Hormones: A Study of Vegetarian and Nonvegetarian Postmenopausal Women." *Journal of the National Cancer Institute* 67, no. 4(1981):761–767.

Avis, N. E., P. A. Kaufert, M. Lock, et al. "The Evolution of Menopausal Symptoms." *Bailliere's Clinical Endocrinology and Metabolism* 7, no. 1(1993):17–33.

Baggott, J. E., T. Ha, W. H. Vaughn, et al. "Effect of Miso (Japanese Soybean Paste) and NaC1 on DMBA-Induced Rat Mammary Tumors." *Nutrition and Cancer* 14(1990): 103–109.

Barnes, S., C. Grubbs, K. D. R. Setchell, and J. Carlson. "Soybeans Inhibit Mammary Tumors in Models of Breast Cancer." *Mutagens and Carcinogens in the Diet* (1990):239–253.

Barnes, S., C. Grubbs, and K. D. R. Setchall. "Chemoprevention by Powdered Soybean Chips (PSC) of Mammary Tumors in Rats." *Breast Cancer Research and Treatment* 12, Abstracts (1988):128.

Benjamin, H., J. Storkson, A. Nagahara, and M. W. Pariza. "Inhibition of Benzo(a)pyrene-induced Mouse Forestomach Neoplasia by Dietary Soy Sauce." *Cancer Research* 51(1991):2940–2942.

Buckley, N. D., and S. A. Carlsen. "Involvement of Soybean Agglutinin-Binding Cells in the Lymphatic Metastasis of the R3230AC Rat Mammary Adenocarcinoma." *Cancer Research* 48(1988):1451–1455.

Campbell, D. R., and M. S. Kurzer. "Flavonoid Inhibition of Aromatase Enzyme Activity in Human Preadipocytes." *Journal of Steroid Biochemistry and Molecular Biology* 46, no. 3(1993):381–388.

Carroll, K. K. "Review of Clinical Studies on Cholesterol-Lowering Response to Soy Protein." *Journal of the American Dietetic Association* 91(1991):820–827.

Carroll, K. K., P. M. Giovannetti, M. W. Huff, et al. "Hypocholesterolemic Effect of Substituting Soybean Protein for Animal Protein in the Diet of Healthy Young Women." *American Journal of Clinical Nutrition* 31(1978):1312–1321.

Coward, L., N. C. Barnes, K. D. R. Setchell, and S. Barnes. "Genistein, Daidzein, and Their β-Glycoside Conjugates: Antitumor Isoflavones in Soybean Foods From American and Asian Diets." *Journal of Agriculture and Food Chemistry* 41(1993):1961–1967.

Dragsted, L.O., M. Strube, and J. C. Larsen. "Cancer Protective Factors in Fruits and Vegetables: Biochemical and Biological Background." *Pharmacology and Toxicology* 72, no. 1, Supplement (1993):116–s.135.

Erdman, J. W., and E. J. Fordyce. "Soy Products and the Human Diet." *American Journal of Clinical Nutrition* 49(1989):725-737.

Farnsworth, N. R., A. S. Bingel, G. A. Cordell, et al. "Potential Value of Plants as Sources of New Antifertility Agents II." *Journal of Pharmaceutical Sciences* 64, no. 5(1975):717–754.

Furukawa, F., K. Imaida, T. Imazawa, et al. "Modifying Effects of Soybean Trypsin Inhibitor on Development of Eosinophilic Nodules and Basophilic Foci in the Exocrine Pancreas of Male Sprague-Dawley Rats Treated with 4-Hydroxyaminoquinoline 1-Oxide." *Japanese Journal of Cancer Research* 83(1992):40–44.

Giovannucci, E., E. B. Rimm, G. A. Colditz, et al. "A Prospective Study of Dietary Fat and Risk of Prostate Cancer." *Journal of the National Cancer Institute* 85, no. 19(1993): 1571–1579.

Goldberg, A. P., A. Lim, J. B. Kolar, et al. "Soybean Protein Independently Lowers Plasma Cholesterol Levels in Primary Hypercholesterolemia." *Atherosclerosis* 43(1982): 355–368.

Golden, B. R., H. Adlercreutz, S. L. Gorbach, et al. "The Relationship Between Estrogen Levels and Diets of Caucasian American and Oriental Immigrant Women." *American Journal of Clinical Nutrition* 44(1986):945–953.

Goodman, M. J., C. J. Stewart, and F. Gilbert. "Patterns of Menopause: A Study of Certain Medical and Physiological Variables Among Caucasian and Japanese Women Living in Hawaii." *Journal of Gerontology* 32, no. 3(1977):291–298.

Goodman, M. J., R. D. Bulbrook, and J. W. Moore. "The Distribution of Estradiol in the Sera of Normal Caucasian, Chinese, Filipina, Hawaiian and Japanese Women Living in Hawaii." *European Journal of Cancer and Clinical Oncology* 24, no. 12(1988):1855–1860.

Graf, E., and J. W. Eaton. "Antioxidant Functions of Phytic Acid." *Free Radical Biology and Medicine* 8(1990):61–69.

Hasdai, A., and I. E. Liener. "The Failure of Long-Term Feeding of Raw Soy Flour, in the Presence or Absence of Azaserine to Induce Carcinogenic Changes in the Mouse Pancreas." *Nutrition and Cancer* 8(1986):85–91.

Hirohata, T., A. M. Y. Nomura, J. H. Hankin, et al. "An Epidemiologic Study on the Association Between Diet and Breast Cancer." *Journal of the National Cancer Institute* 78, no. 1(1987):595–600.

Hughes, C. L. "Phytochemical Mimicry of Reproductive Hormones and Modulation of Herbivore Fertility by Phytoestrogens." *Enviromental Health Perspectives* 78:(1988) 171–175.

Jariwalla, R. J., R. Sabin, S. Lawson, et al. "Effects of Dietary Phytic Acid (Phytate) on the Incidence and Growth Rate of Tumors Promoted in Fischer Rats by a Magnesium Supplement." *Nutrition Research* 8(1988):813–827.

Jenkins, D. J. A., T. M. S. Wolever, G. Spiller, et al. "Hypocholesterolemic Effect of Vegetable Protein in a Hypocaloric Diet." *Atherosclerosis* 78(1989)78:99–107.

Jirtle, R. L., J. D. Haag, E. A. Ariazi, and M. N. Gould. "Increased Mannose 6-Phosphate/Insulin-Like Growth-Factor II Receptor and Transforming Growth Factor β1 Levels During Monoterpene-Induced Regression of Mammary Tumors." *Cancer Research* 53(1993):3849–3852.

Kaldas, R. S., and C. L. Hughes. "Reproductive and General Metabolic Effects of Phytoestrogens in Mammals." *Reproductive Toxicology* 3(1989):81–89.

Kanazawa, T., M. Tanaka, U. Tsugumichi, et al. "Anti-atherogenicity of Soybean Protein." *Annals of New York Academy of Science* 676(1993):202–214.

Kennedy, A. R., P. C. Billings, P. A. Maki, and P. Newberne. "Effects of Various Preparations of Dietary Protease Inhibitors on Oral Carcinogenesis in Hamsters Induced by DMBA." *Nutrition and Cancer* 19(1993):191–200.

Kune, G. A., S. Bannerman, B. Field, et al. "Diet, Alcohol, Smoking, Serum β-Carotene and Vitamin A in Male Non-melanocytic Skin Cancer Patients and Controls." *Nutrition and Cancer* 18(1992):237–244.

Lee, H. P., L. Gourley, S. W. Duffy, et al. "Dietary Effects on Breast-Cancer Risk in Singapore." *The Lancet* 337 (May 18, 1991):1197–1200.

Lee, I. M., J. E. Manson, C. H. Hennekens, and R. S. Paffenbarger. "Body Weight and Mortality: a 27-Year Follow-up of Middle-Aged Men." *Journal of the American Medical Association* 270(1993):2823–2828.

Librenti, M. C., M. Cocchi, E. Orsi, et al. "Effect of Soya and Cellulose Fibers on Postprandial Glycemic Response in Type II Diabetic Patients." *Diabetes Care* 15, no. 1(1992): 111–113.

Lo, G. S. "Physiological Effects and Physico-Chemical Properties of Soy Cotyledon Fiber." *Advances in Experimental Medicine and Biology* 270(1990):49–66.

Lo, G. S., A. P. Goldberg, A. Lim, et al. "Soy Fiber Improves Lipid and Carbohydrate Metabolism in Primary Hyperlipidemic Subjects." *Atherosclerosis* 62(1986):239–248.

Lock, M. "Ambiguities of Aging: Japanese Experience and Perceptions of Menopause." *Culture, Medicine and Psychiatry* 10(1986):23–46.

Lock, M., P. Kaufert, and P. Gilbert. "Cultural Construction of the Menopausal Syndrome: the Japanese Case." *Maturitas* 10(1988):317–332.

Loy, T. S., J. Kyle, and J. T. Bickel. "Binding of Soybean Agglutinin Lectin to Prostatic Hyperplasia and Adenocarcinoma." *Cancer* 63(1989):1583–1586.

Madar, Z. "Effect of Brown Rice and Soybean Dietary Fiber on the Control of Glucose and Lipid Metabolism in Diabetic Rats." *American Journal of Clinical Nutrition* 38(1983): 388–393.

Maeda, H., T. Katsuki, T. Akaike, and R. Yasutake. "High Correlation Between Lipid Peroxide Radical and Tumor Promoter Effect: Suppression of Tumor Promotion in the Epstein-Barr Virus/B-Lymphocyte System and Scavenging of Alkyl Peroxide Radicals by Various Vegetable Extracts." *Japanese Journal of Cancer Research* 83(1992):923–928.

Martin, P. M., K. B. Horwitz, D. S. Ryan, and W. L. McGuire. "Phytoestrogen Interaction with Estrogen Receptors in Human Breast Cancer Cells." *Endocrinology* 103, no. 5(1978):1860–1867.

Matsukawa, Y., N. Marui, T. Sakai, et al. "Genistein Arrests Cell Cycle Progression at G_2-M." *Cancer Research* 53 (March 15, 1993):1328–1331.

McGuinness, E. E., R. G. H. Morgan, and K. G. Wormsely.

"Effects of Soybean Flour on the Pancreas of Rats." *Environmental Health Perspectives* 56(1984):205–212.

Messina, M., and S. Barnes. "The Role of Soy Products in Reducing Risk of Cancer." *Journal of the National Cancer Institute* 83, no. 8(1991):541–546.

Messina, M., and V. Messina. "Increasing Use of Soyfoods and Their Potential Role in Cancer Prevention." *Journal of the American Dietetic Association* 91(1991):836–840.

Meydani, S. N., A. H. Lichtenstein, P. J. White, et al. "Food Use and Health Effects of Soybean and Sunflower Oils." *Journal of the American College of Nutrition* 10, no. 5(1991): 406–428.

Miksicek, R. J. "Commonly Occuring Plant Flavonoids Have Estrogenic Activity." *Molecular Pharmacology* 44(1993): 37–43.

Mokhtar, N. M., A. A. El-Asser, M. N. El-Bolkainy, et al. "Effect of Soybean Feeding on Experimental Carcinogenesis-III. Carcinogenecity of Nitrite and Dibutylamine in Mice: a Histopathological Study." *European Journal of Cancer and Clinical Oncology* 24, no. 3(1988):403–411.

Moore, J. W., G. M. G. Clark, O. Takatani, et al. "Distribution of 17 β-Estradiol in the Sera of Normal British and Japanese Women." *Journal of the National Cancer Institute* 71, no. 4(1983):749–754.

Nomura, A., B. E. Henderson, and J. Lee. "Breast Cancer and Diet Among the Japanese in Hawaii." *American Journal of Clinical Nutrition* 31(1978):2020–2025.

Peterson, G., and S. Barnes. "Genistein and Biochanin A Inhibit the Growth of Human Prostate Cancer Cells but Not Epidermal Growth Factor Receptor Tyrosine Autophosphorylation." *The Prostate* 22(1993):335–345.

Peterson, G., and S. Barnes. "Genistein Inhibition of the Growth of Human Breast Cancer Cells: Independence From Estrogen Receptors and the Multi-Drug Resistance Chain." *Biochemical and Biophysical Research Communications* 179, no. 1(1991):661–667.

Phipps, W. R., M. C. Martini, J. W. Lampe, et al. "Effect of Flax

Seed Ingestion on the Menstrual Cycle." *Journal of Clinical Endocrinology and Metabolism* 77, no. 5(1993):1215–1219.

Reese, M. R., and D. A. Chow. "Tumor Progression *in Vivo*: Increased Soybean Agglutinin Lectin Binding, *N*-Acetyl-galactosamine-Specific Lectin Expression, and Liver Metastasis Potential." *Cancer Research* 52(1992):5235–5243.

Rose, D. P. "Diet, Hormones and Cancer." *Annual Review of Public Health* 14(1993):1–17.

Rose, D. P. "Dietary Fiber, Phytoestrogens, and Breast Cancer." *Nutrition* 8, no. 1 (January-February 1992):47–51.

Rosenberger, N. "Menopause as a Symbol of Anomaly: the Case of Japanese Women." *Health Care For Women International* 7, no. 1–2(1986):15–24.

Salerno, J. W., and D. E. Smith. "The Use of Sesame Oil and Other Vegetable Oils in the Inhibition of Human Colon Cancer Growth *in Vitro*." *Anticancer Research* 2(1991):209–216.

Setchell, K. D. R., S. P. Borriello, P. Hulme, et al. "Nonsteroidal Estrogens of Dietary Origin: Possible Role in Hormone-Dependent Disease." *American Journal of Clinical Nutrition* 40(1984):568–578.

Sharma, O. P., H. Adlercreutz, J. D. Strandberg, et al. "Soy of Dietary Source Plays a Preventive Role Against the Pathogenesis of Prostatitis in Rats." *Journal of Steroid Biochemistry and Molecular Biology* 43, no. 6(1992):557–564.

Shimizu, H., R. K. Ross, L. Bernstein, et al. "Serum Oestrogen Levels in Postmenopausal Women: Comparison of American Whites and Japanese in Japan." *British Journal of Cancer* 62(1990):451–453.

Sirtori, C. R., C. Zucchi-Dentone, M. Sitori, et al. "Cholesterol-Lowering and HDL-Raising Properties of Lecithinated Soy Proteins in Type II Hyperlipidemic Patients." *Annals of Nutrition and Metabolism* 29(1985):348–357.

Sirtori, C. R., E. Gatti, O. Mantero, et al. "Clinical Experience With the Soybean Protein Diet in the Treatment of Hypercholesterolemia." *American Journal of Clinical Nutrition* 32(1979):1645–1658.

Sirtori, C. R., E. Agradi, F. Conti, et al. "Soybean-Protein Diet in the Treatment of Type-II Hyperlipoproteinaemia." *The Lancet* (February 5, 1977):275–277.

Slavin, J. "Nutritional Benefits of Soy Protein and Soy Fiber." *Journal of the American Dietetic Association* 91(1991):816–819.

Soda, M. Y., H. Mizunuma, S. I. Honjo, et al. "Pre- and Post-menopausal Bone Mineral Density of the Spine and Proximal Femur in Japanese Women Assessed by Dual-Energy X-Ray Absorptiometry: A Cross-Sectional Study." *Journal of Bone and Mineral Research* 8, no. 2(1993):183–189.

Söderström, K. O., "Lectin Binding to Prostatic Adenocarcinoma." *Cancer* 60(1987):1823–1831.

St. Clair, W. H., P. C. Billings, J. A. Carew, et al. "Suppression of Dimethylhydrazine-Induced Carcinogenesis in Mice by Dietary Addition of the Bowman-Birk Protease Inhibitor." *Cancer Research* 50(1990):580–586.

Takatani, O., H. Kosano, T. Okumoto, et al. "Distribution of Estradiol and Percentage of Free Testosterone in Sera of Japanese Women: Preoperative Breast Cancer Patients and Normal Controls." *Journal of the National Cancer Institute* 79, no. 6(1987)1199–1204.

Teas, J. "The Consumption of Seaweed as a Protective Factor in the Etiology of Breast Cancer." *Medical Hypotheses* 7(1981):601–613.

Traganos, F., B. Ardelt, H. Halko, et al. "Effects of Genistein on the Growth and Cell Cycle Progression of Normal Human Lymphocytes and Human Leukemic MOLT-4 and HL-60 Cells." *Cancer Research* 52(1992):6200–6208.

Trichopoulos, D., S. Yen, J. Brown, et al. "The Effect of Westernization on Urine Estrogens, Frequency of Ovulation, and Breast Cancer Risk: a Study of Ethnic Chinese Women in the Orient and the USA." *Cancer* 53(1984):187–192.

Troll, W., and A. R. Kennedy (eds.). "Meeting Report: Workshop Report From the Division of Cancer Etiology, National Cancer Institute, National Institutes of Health: Protease Inhibitors as Cancer Chemopreventive Agents." *Cancer Research* 49(1989):499–502.

Troll, W., R. Wiesner, C. J. Shellabarger, et al. "Soybean Diet Lowers Breast Tumor Incidence in Irradiated Rats." *Carcinogenesis* 1(1980):469–472.

Tuyns, A. J., R. Kaaks, and M. Haelterman. "Colorectal Cancer and the Consumption of Foods: A Case Control Study in Belgium." *Nutrition and Cancer* 11(1988):189–204.

Ushiroyama, T., Y. Okamoto, and O. Sugimoto. "Plasma Lipid and Lipoprotein Levels in Perimenopausal Women." *Acta Obstetricia et Gynecologica Scandinavica* 72(1993):428–433.

Verrillo, A., A. de Teresa, P. C. Giarrusso, and S. La Rocca. "Soybean Protein Diets in the Management of Type II Hyperlipoproteinaemia." *Atherosclerosis* 54(1985):321–331.

Vucenik, I., V. J. Tomzaic, D. Fabian, and A. M. Shamsuddin. "Antitumor Activity of Phytic Acid (Inositol Hexaphosphate) in Murine Tansplanted and Metastatic Fibrosarcoma, a Pilot Study." *Cancer Letters* 65(1992):9–13.

Watanabe, H., T. Okamoto, T. Takahashi, et al. "The Effects of Sodium Chloride, Miso or Ethanol on Development of Intestinal Metaplasia After X-Irradiation of the Rat Glandular Stomach." *Japanese Journal of Cancer Research* 83(1992):1267–1272.

Webb, T. E., P. C. Stomberg, H. Abou-Issa, et al. "Effect of Dietary Soybean and Licorice on the Male F344 Rat: An Integrated Study of Some Parameters Relevant to Cancer Chemoprevention." *Nutrition and Cancer* 18(1992):215–230.

Weed, H. G., R. B. McGandy, and A. R. Kennedy. "Protection Against Dimethylhydrazine-Induced Adenomatous Tumors of the Mouse Color by the Dietary Addition of an Extract of Soybeans Containing the Bowman-Birk Protease Inhibitor." *Carcinogenesis* 6, no. 8(1985):1239–1241.

Welshons, W. V., C. S. Murphy, R. Koch, et al. "Stimulation of Breast Cancer Cells *in Vitro* by the Environmental Estrogen Enterolactone and the Phytoestrogen Equol." *Breast Cancer Research and Treatment* 10(1987):169–175.

Wilcox, G., M. L. Wahlqvist, H. G. Burger, and G. Medley. "Oestrogenic Effects of Plant Foods in Postmenopausal Women." *British Medical Journal* 301(1990):905–906.

Yavelow, J., T. H. Finlay, A. R. Kennedy, and W. Troll. "Bowman-Birk Soybean Protease Inhibitor as an Anticarcinogen." *Cancer Research* 43, Supplement (1983):2454s–2459s.

Index

EARL MINDELL IS ALSO THE AUTHOR OF:

Earl Mindell's Herb Bible

Earl Mindell's Food as Medicine

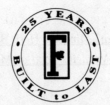